pocket
calorie
counter

pocket
calorie
counter

carolyn humphries

foulsham
LONDON • NEW YORK • TORONTO • SYDNEY

foulsham

Capital Point, 33 Bath Road, Slough, Berkshire, SL1 3UF, England

Foulsham books can be found in all good bookshops and direct from www.foulsham.com

ISBN 978-0-572-03427-6

Copyright © 2008 W. Foulsham & Co. Ltd
Last reprinted 2011

Neither the editors of W. Foulsham & Co. Ltd nor the author nor the publisher take responsibility for any possible consequences from any procedure, test, exercise or action by any person reading or following the information in this book. The publication of this book does not constitute the practice of medicine, and this book does not attempt to replace any diet or instructions from your doctor. The author and publisher advise the reader to check with a doctor before starting a diet, administering any medication or undertaking any course of treatment or exercise.

Printed in Great Britain by Martins the Printers Ltd, Berwick upon Tweed.

Contents

Introduction

There are lots of calorie counters in the bookshops, but this one is, I think, genuinely different – and much better. Before starting to write it, I thought very carefully about how you want to use a calorie counter. Having looked at those already on offer, I asked myself some questions.

- Is it useful to have to search under obscure brand names where you can't find things and can't compare them easily with similar products? No!
- Do you want to work out what category a food belongs to before you try to find it? Hardly likely.
- Do you really have time to worry that one Rich Tea biscuit has four more calories than another? I don't think so.
- Is it helpful to tell you the calories per 100 g, leaving you to work out how much you are eating and how many calories it contains? Do you really want to

carry a kitchen scales and a calculator when you're going to meet your friends in that hot new café? Life's too short!

With this handy little book you can forget all of those problems, because it gives you the real essentials, uniquely organised and calculated to make everything easy. It tells you how many calories you are consuming in everything you eat, from breakfast through to dinner – every snack and every drink, at home or eating out.

Most people who use this book will be doing so because they want to lose weight, but you can also use it if you want to gain weight. It may be small, but this at-a-glance calorie counter has all the information you need to achieve and maintain a healthy lifestyle, including great tips that really will make dieting easy.

A Healthy Lifestyle

Dieting of any kind, whether to lose or gain weight, should be part of a healthy lifestyle. Crank dieting is stupid and it doesn't work. If you try to lose weight by cutting out a particular food group, you may succeed, but you'll also become unfit and possibly even ill. In the same way, if you are trying to gain weight, eating mountains of sugary and fatty foods is not the answer.

Your body needs nutrients containing vitamins and minerals as well as the proper balance of protein, carbohydrate, fat and fibre to keep you fit and healthy. So as well as the calories, you need to choose a balanced diet containing foods from all the main food groups, maximising fruits and vegetables and minimising processed foods and foods that contain high amounts of sugar, salt and fat.

Carbohydrates

It may surprise you to know that complex carbohydrates, or starchy foods, should make up 50 per cent of each of your meals. This is because carbohydrates provide us with energy and are vital to our well-being. However, the added sugar (simple carbohydrates) and fat you mix with them will pile on the unwanted calories that can harm your health. The best sources of complex carbohydrates are bread (all types, but wholemeal is the most nutritious), pasta, rice, cereals (this includes breakfast cereals but you should choose wholegrain varieties not sugar-coated ones) and potatoes. Eat plenty of all of these.

Fat

You do need some fat in your diet – but not too much – to provide body warmth and energy. Fat is also essential for proper brain function. There is enough for your daily needs contained naturally in foods so keep added fat to a minimum and eat it sparingly (see my Clever diet tips for losing weight on pages 26–27).

Fibre

Your body also needs fibre – it is particularly necessary for your digestive function. You should eat plenty of fruit and vegetables, wholegrains, and the skins on potatoes.

Proteins

Your body needs protein to maintain good health and to repair itself when necessary. The best sources of proteins are fish, lean meat, poultry, dairy products, eggs and vegetable proteins such as pulses (dried peas, beans and lentils), tofu and Quorn. Eat two to three small portions a day.

Vitamins and minerals

These are also essential for general good health. A balanced diet of fresh foods from all the main food groups should contain sufficient vitamins and minerals to keep your body healthy, and supplements should not be necessary for the vast majority of people.

The best sources are fruit and vegetables. They should, preferably, be fresh, but frozen or canned in water or natural juice with no added sugar (and, ideally, no added salt) are fine. Eat at least five portions a day.

Liquids

You also need lots of liquid in your diet. Make sure you drink plenty of water – from the tap, filtered or mineral according to your preference. If you're really not keen on water, flavour it with a low-calorie squash.

Pure fruit juices are good for you and count as one portion of your five-a-day fruit and vegetables (however much you drink). The vitamin C in them helps you absorb the iron in foods such as fortified breakfast cereals too. Fruit drinks do contain calories, however, so they must be counted in your daily allowance.

Tea and coffee may be drunk in moderation but preferably after or between meals, as the tannin in the beverages impairs the absorption of some essential nutrients. If you want to add milk, use skimmed or semi-skimmed. Alternatively, drink both tea and coffee black (tea with lemon is deliciously refreshing and contains hardly any calories). Don't add any sugar. If you have a sweet tooth, use artificial sweeteners, but, ideally, wean yourself off them. Learning to do without sweetness will help your new, healthy lifestyle.

Try to consume at least 300 ml/½ pt/1¼ cups of skimmed or semi-skimmed milk during the day; this includes what you put on cereal or use in cooking. If you have a lot of weight to lose, then go for the skimmed option.

Alcohol

Alcohol is not a dieter's friend. If you are trying to lose weight, it piles on 'empty' calories, so have it as a treat only. Use low-calorie mixers with spirits and go for low-strength beers. If you like wine, try having a spritzer (wine diluted with sparkling water). Whatever you do, don't use drink as a substitute for good, nutritious food.

Regular exercise

An active body is more likely to be a healthy body. However, one mad burst of exercise a week at the gym isn't a good idea (although it's better than nothing). You need to take more frequent, regular exercise to reap the benefit.

There are plenty of ways to exercise without jogging or work-outs. Get into the habit of walking briskly instead of wandering along. Go on foot whenever possible instead of using the car or public transport. If you take the bus, get off a stop before your usual one and walk the last part of the journey. Ride a bike if you have one. Use the stairs instead of lifts or escalators. Take up a recreational sport like tennis or swimming or join an activity like a dance class. Even energetic gardening will burn off calories.

Bending and stretching exercises will also help to tone your muscles but seek advice before you start any exercise regime – you must do them correctly or you can cause injury. If you are going to do exercises at home, do them at a fixed time, perhaps as soon as you get out of bed or before you have your shower or bath in the morning or evening. Try to make them a regular part of your daily routine, otherwise the novelty will wear off after a few days and you won't persevere.

Controlling Your Weight

Calorie counting is an efficient way of controlling your diet and so adjusting your weight. To lose weight, your energy, or calorie, intake from food and drink (that's the calories in the food you eat) needs to be less than your energy output (the number of calories you burn up through activity). Strictly speaking, the measure we refer to as 'calories' should actually be called kilocalories (units of 1,000 calories) but they are always abbreviated to kcalories, or calories.

An average man uses about 2,500 calories a day; a woman about 1,900 calories. The difference is partly because of size and partly because women tend to have a slower metabolic rate – they don't use up calories as quickly as men. The more active your lifestyle and the more exercise you undertake, the more calories you will use up.

If you only want to lose a small amount of weight and you want to do it fairly quickly, you should aim for a low daily calorie intake – say 1,500 calories for a man, 1,000 calories for a woman. But if you are planning a long-term, substantial weight reduction, it is much more effective to take it more slowly, aiming at, say, 1,900 calories per day for a man and 1,500 for a woman.

If you are underweight, of course, you will need to consume more calories than you burn in order to gain weight. Again, slow and steady is the way to go.

Your perfect weight

It is crucial that you are realistic about the weight you want to be. Having established the weight that you are aiming for, you should plan for a slow and steady weight loss, or gain, and work towards maintaining a healthy, balanced diet as your normal routine.

Below is a chart, based on UK government statistics (for adults only), which shows you how much you should weigh according to your height. Your bone structure will dictate whether you are at the lower end of the scale or higher up. The important thing is to be within the limits of your ideal weight.

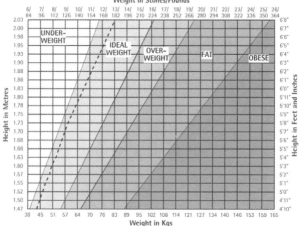

Weigh yourself first thing in the morning, preferably without clothes. If you weigh yourself when you are dressed, make sure you are wearing similar clothing each time. Check where you are on the table, then work out how much weight you need to lose or gain.

Once you've made that calculation and started your diet, weigh yourself on the same scales, in the same way, once a week only. Avoid the temptation to keep hopping on and off the scales, as weight fluctuates throughout the day and from day to day, which will only make you disheartened. There is usually a quick burst of weight loss in the first few days of a slimming diet, then the rate of loss will level off. Weighing yourself once a week will give you a much clearer picture of your progress. In the same way, if you are trying to put on weight, there may be an initial burst, then your weight will reach a plateau for a while before rising again.

Don't give up. If you are following a healthy and sensible balanced diet, you will be rewarded in the end.

Calories and exercise

Regular exercise doesn't just burn up calories, it is a vital part of a healthy lifestyle. You'll see from this list (which is based on a woman of average height and build) the difference between the number of calories you use up doing physically active tasks and the more leisurely ones.

Activity	Calories used in 30 minutes	Activity	Calories used in 30 minutes
Aerobics	210	House work	120
Ballroom dancing	190	Jogging	165
Climbing stairs	330	Manual work, heavy	225
Cycling, fast or uphill	330	Manual work, light	120
Cycling, leisurely speed	120	Running, fast	200
Disco dancing	205	Shopping	120
Driving a car	60	Sleeping	30
Gardening, digging	240	Squash	273
Gardening, hoeing	105	Swimming, racing speed	300
Golf	195	Swimming, relaxed speed	255
Gym work-out	210	Tennis	250
Hill-walking	240	Typing	60
Horse-riding, hacking	60	Walking, relaxed speed	120
Horse-riding, trotting and cantering	180	Walking, briskly	180
		Watching TV	45

Planning your diet

To keep a strict note of your calorie intake, you need to plan your day's menu, including drinks. Then look up each item and add the calorie totals together. The full amount should be equal to or less than your limit to lose weight; if you wish to gain weight, it should be above your limit. If the result is lower than your planned count for the day, you can give yourself an extra snack or another portion of healthy food, such as a vegetable or some bread with your meal. If you're over the limit and on a reducing diet, then you must find a lower-calorie alternative, perhaps grilled (broiled) fish instead of a fish pie, or fruit salad instead of apple crumble. To help you reduce your calorie count without even realising, I have included some cunning diet tips on pages 26–29.

Do read the tips for a healthy lifestyle on page 9, too. If you want your diet to work long-term and to keep fit and well, it is essential that you follow a sensible, balanced diet.

Going out for a meal

If you are trying to lose weight and you are invited out for a meal, don't panic. Most of the dishes you're likely to come across are in this book – even down to your aperitif or glass of wine. However, don't let yourself become a bore about it. Other people around you won't be dieting and if they see you constantly poring over your little guide, they will think you're obsessive. It's probably better to consult the book before you go out – you will soon get to know what are low-calorie foods and what are the blow-outs. Stick to the goodies if you can, but if you can't, don't worry. If you go over your calorie limit one day, then make sure the next day you stay under your limit by a similar amount to even out your average daily intake. But be warned, this will only work if you do it on an occasional basis. You can't expect to be able to cheat all the time. It's pointless to keep going over your limit, telling yourself that tomorrow you'll be good. Try to stick to your calorie limit every day, or you won't see the benefits.

Diet and health foods

There are many ranges of special diet foods available. They are relatively expensive, however, and do not offer any guarantee that you will actually lose weight. That said, low-calorie options can be useful when you are controlling your calories.

Regulations governing food labelling mean that the word 'diet' can appear on a label only if the food is a low-calorie one. In order to be so-named, it must contain no more than 40 calories per 100 g/4 oz or 100 ml/3½ fl oz and must state clearly that it can only help weight loss if consumed as part of a calorie-controlled diet.

Many foods claim to be nutritionally 'better for you' and there are voluntary guidelines in place over what some of these definitions mean. However, they can be rather vague, and some of the products that make this claim may be no better than the standard product. The only way to be sure is to read the labels (and this book!) and see the nutritional values for yourself. Overleaf is a guide to what the wording on the labels means.

Fat-free
Contains no more than 0.15 g of fat per 100 g.

Low in saturates
Contains no more than 3 per cent saturated fat per 100 g.

Sugar-free
Contains no more than 0.2 g of sugar per 100 g.

No added sugar
Has no sugar or foods made up mainly of sugars (e.g. dried fruit or concentrated fruit juice) added to it or any of its ingredients.

Reduced fat/reduced sugar
Contains at least 25 per cent less fat/sugar than the standard product.

High fibre
Contains more than 6 g fibre per 100 g.

Low fat/low sugar
Contains no more than 5 g fat/sugar per 100 g.

Low sodium
Contains no more than 40 mg sodium per 100 g.

All of the above are fairly clear. But there are other terms, commonly used on labels, that are not covered by the guidelines, and these can be more ambiguous.

Lower fat
This means the food has less fat than the standard product, but that may be a high-fat product and the quantity may only be reduced by a tiny fraction!

Light or lite
This is likely to mean lower in fat but it could mean lighter in weight, colour, or even texture! These, and lower fat foods, may have more sugar and starch (so more calories) to make them taste better.

Virtually fat-free
This should mean the food contains very little fat and so is a good one to look out for. But see below.

90 per cent fat-free
Sounds good – but in reality it means the product contains 10 per cent fat. This means it has more fat than one labelled 'low-fat'!

Clever diet tips for losing weight

You don't have to go on a special diet to lose weight – there are lots of ways to cut down on the calories whilst continuing to eat normal meals.

- Choose low-fat yoghurts, cheeses, cream, etc.
- Drink skimmed milk.
- Beware of cream substitutes – they often have more calories than the real thing!
- Fill up on as many vegetables or salad stuffs as you like – as long as they are not laced with gallons of oil or melted butter!
- Remove all of the fat or skin from meat and poultry before eating.
- Choose lean meats and always trim off any excess fat before cooking.
- Grill (broil) rather than fry.
- Use a low-fat spread instead of butter and add only a scraping to bread. Don't add any extra to vegetables before serving. I have given the calorie

count for an average spreading in the book. If you can use half that amount, do so. (You will reap the benefits in reduced calories!)

- Beware of spread or butter melting into hot toast and 'clumping' on new bread – you won't be able to resist adding more!
- Use only the minimum of oil for cooking and drain off any excess.
- When browning meat for a made-up dish, dry-fry rather than adding oil and spoon off any fat.
- Don't add sugar to fruits, cereals or drinks.
- Choose low-calorie brands of drinks, dressings, etc.
- Drink plenty of water.
- Choose fruits canned in natural juice only, not syrup, and drink unsweetened pure juices. Beware of cartons labelled as fruit juice 'drinks' – these contain sugar and other additives.

Tips to make losing weight easier

Simply reducing the quantity of food you eat will help greatly in cutting down your calorie intake. If you are normally used to eating very large portions, try any of the following.

- Use a smaller plate for meals.
- A glass of naturally sparkling mineral water with your meal will help fill you up. Drink it in between meals too – zip it up with a slice of lemon or lime.
- Use a strong-flavoured cheese when cooking. You won't need to add so much to give it a good flavour.
- Cut foods into smaller pieces or thinner slices and serve yourself your usual number of pieces/slices – you'll think you've had the same but you'll actually have had less.
- Keep your butter or other spread at room temperature. It will spread much more easily, so you will use much less and save lots of calories. For example, a slice of bread and butter is 169 calories,

but spread thinly with warm butter it will be only 132 calories!

- Chew slowly and eat small forkfuls. Your meal will last longer, giving you time to feel more satisfied.
- Never go shopping on an empty stomach – it's far too tempting.
- Try to eat meals before you're ravenously hungry – especially if you are going to a restaurant!
- If you go out for a meal, don't skip the starter in the hope that you'll save calories. Opt for a low-calorie one – together with the main course it will take the edge off your appetite, and with any luck you'll be able to avoid the calorie-packed desserts!
- If you feel really peckish, eat some raw carrots – or any salad vegetables, or a bunch of grapes or a few slices of apple – to keep you going and take the edge off your appetite.
- Make a drink of meat or yeast extract (such as Bovril or Marmite) – a teaspoon in a mug of boiling water. It will take the edge off your appetite and help to fill you up between meals.

- Keep a packet of sugar-free chewing gum handy and chew between meals. Alternatively, clean your teeth instead of grabbing a snack – it really works!
- Always take the trouble to make your meal look appetising. A sprinkling of parsley or vegetables attractively arranged can help you really enjoy what's on your plate rather than just eating for the sake of it.
- Don't cheat! You know if you are piling food on your plate so try to be less-than-generous. Just remember, the smaller the portion, the more you'll lose. Average portion means average, not piled high!
- Don't weigh yourself more than once a week.

How to Use this Book

Using the book is simplicity itself. You will find everything from a slice of bread to a Tournedos rossini in here, and they are all easy to find.

- All the foods are listed alphabetically so that you can find them easily without having to work out a category or recall an obscure name.
- Columns are clearly marked and there are dictionary-style page headings so you can easily flick through to the place you want to find.
- All the calories given are per portion, so you don't have anything to work out. It even gives you the average calories for made-up dishes, so you don't have to weigh or calculate a thing.
- The amount of carbohydrate and fat is listed for every item, plus a measure of the fibre content.

- If something may be found under two different names, I have included them under both and cross-referenced them.
- Prepared meals can be found under both the initial letter of the recipe title and also under the main ingredient. So Tandoori chicken may be found under both T for tandoori and C for chicken.
- Where a product has different variations, I have listed it under its generic name. So, for example, you'll find all the varieties of milk under M: 'Milk, skimmed', 'Milk, semi-skimmed' and so on.
- Where a food has different flavours, as do crisps (potato chips), for example, I have given an average calorie content for all the flavours. You can always check the specific food labels for the exact calorie count, but the difference is only one or two calories!

Portion sizes

To make the book really dieter-friendly, I have calculated the foods using average portions. To be sure of success with your diet, you must stick to these portion sizes. To make it clearer still – and harder for you to cheat – the table below explains exactly what I mean by each portion size. If you give yourself larger portions, you will suffer the consequences!

Food	Portion size given	Equivalent weight or size
Butter or other spreads	1 small knob	10 g/¼ oz/2 tsp
Cakes and pies	1 slice	⅛ of a standard pie or cake ⅙ large pizza or quiche
Cereals These vary according to type (flakes, porridge, etc.) and are based on manufacturer's recommended serving size. Use a large serving spoon, not a measuring spoon.	3 heaped tablespoons 5 heaped tablespoons	50 g or 40 g 40 g or 30 g
Cheese	1 small wedge/1 good spoonful/1 small chunk	25 g/1 oz

Food	Portion size given	Equivalent weight or size
Chocolate	1 standard bar	One size up from fun size. (The standard bars vary but are on average around 40 g.)
Drinks	1 small (beer/cider)	300 ml/½ pt/1¼ cups
	1 small glass	100 ml/3½ fl oz/scant ½ cup
	1 wine glass	120 ml/4 fl oz/½ cup
	1 tumbler	200 ml/7 fl oz/scant 1 cup
	1 mug	250 ml/8 fl oz/1 cup
	1 single measure	25 ml/1 fl oz/1½ tbsp
	1 double measure	50 ml/2 fl oz/3 tbsp
Fish	1 (piece of) fillet/1 steak	175 g/6 oz
Fruit and vegetables	3 heaped tablespoons	100 g/4 oz
	2 tablespoons	50 g/2 oz
	1 good handful	Approximately 25 g/1 oz (but it doesn't really matter as the calorie content is tiny!)
Ice cream	1 scoop	50 g/2 oz
Meat and poultry, roast	2 thick slices/3 medium slices/4 thin slices	100 g/4 oz
Sandwiches	1 round	2 medium slices of white bread, spread with butter, plus filling

Food	Portion size given	Equivalent weight or size
Steaks	1 medium steak	175 g/6 oz
	1 large steak (T-bone)	350 g/12 oz
Noodles, all types	1 serving	50 g/2 oz uncooked
Nuts and dried fruit	1 small handful	15 g/½ oz
Pasta, all types	1 serving	75 g/3 oz uncooked
Rice, all types and other grains	1 serving	50 g/2 oz/¼ cup uncooked
Soup	2 ladlefuls	200 ml/7 fl oz/scant 1 cup
	1 mug	250 ml/8 fl oz/1 cup
Sauces and sundries	1 tablespoon	15 ml
	1 teaspoon	5 ml
Snacks	1 small bag	Crisps (chips): 25g
		Corn snacks, chocolate, peanuts, etc: 50 g

Prepared dishes

For prepared dishes, whether home-made or bought ready-prepared, I have referred throughout to the measure '1 serving'. This means one standard, average-sized serving. If the dish is home-made, and the recipe is designed to serve four people, '1 serving' denotes a quarter of the whole dish. In the same way, if a cook-chill or frozen meal is labelled as serving two, '1 serving' will be half the dish. If you eat the whole lot, you must double the calories!

Remember also that recipes vary, so you must be sensible about the content of those you choose. If you know the version you are cooking has loads of extra cream in it, don't kid yourself it is a standard one. When calculating the calorific and nutritional content of each item and recipe, I have estimated the content of an average portion and average recipe.

Brand names

The information has been gathered using both UK and American data. Obviously different brands of a product do not have identical nutritional values and manufacturers change their recipes from time to time, so the figures I have used are averages and may vary slightly from the brands you buy. Always read your labels for the latest and most precise data.

A–Z of Calorie Values

The easy-to-follow page headings and clear presentation mean that you will quickly and easily find the items you are looking for.

You can make your own notes on favourite brands, recipe ideas and food combinations at the end of each section.

Food	kC/ portion	Portion size	Carbs g	Fat g	Fibre
Abbey crunch biscuits (cookies)	**46**	1 biscuit	7	2	low
Absinthe	**55**	1 single measure	trace	trace	0
Ace chocolate bar	**126**	1 standard bar	16	6	low
Aduki beans, dried, soaked and boiled	**123**	3 heaped tbsp	22	trace	high
Advocaat	**68**	1 single measure	7	2	0
Aero chocolate bar, mint	**254**	1 standard bar	28	13	0
Aero chocolate bar, orange	**254**	1 standard bar	28	13	0
Aero chocolate bar, milk	**251**	1 standard bar	26	13	0
Afelia (greek pork stew)	**369**	1 serving	12	28	low
After eight mints	**32**	1 mint	6	1	0
Aioli	**237**	2 tbsp	trace	23	0
Alfalfa sprouts	**7**	1 good handful	1	trace	high
All-bran, dry	**68**	25 g/1 oz/½ cup	11	1	high
All-bran, with semi-skimmed milk	**139**	5 heaped tbsp	16	3	high
All-bran, with skimmed milk	**123**	5 heaped tbsp	16	1	high
Almond biscuits (cookies)	**46**	1 biscuit	6	2	low
Almond danish pastry	**420**	1 pastry	46	24	medium
Almond macaroon	**120**	1 macaroon	13	7	medium
Almond paste	**101**	25 g/1 oz	17	4	medium
Almond slice	**132**	1 slice	21	5	low

Food	kC/ portion	Portion size	Carbs g	Fat g	Fibre
Almonds, fresh, shelled	153	25 g/1 oz/¼ cup	2	14	high
Almonds, ground	46	1 tbsp	trace	4	high
Almonds, roasted	95	1 small handful	1	9	high
Almonds, sugared	15	1 sweet (candy)	3	trace	high
Alpen, dry	91	25 g/1 oz/¼ cup	16	2	high
Alpen, with semi-skimmed milk	203	3 heaped tbsp	33	5	high
Alpen, with skimmed milk	189	3 heaped tbsp	33	3	high
Alpen, no added sugar, dry	89	25 g/1 oz/¼ cup	15	2	high
Alpen, no added sugar, with semi-skimmed milk	200	3 heaped tbsp	31	5	high
Alpen, no added sugar, with skimmed milk	184	3 heaped tbsp	31	3	high
Alpen nutty crunch, dry	95	25 g/1 oz/¼ cup	16	2	high
Alpen nutty crunch, with semi-skimmed milk	209	3 heaped tbsp	32	6	high
Alpen nutty crunch, with skimmed milk	193	3 heaped tbsp	32	4	high
Alphabetti spaghetti, canned	135	1 small can	28	1	medium
Alphabetti spaghetti, on toast	304	1 small can plus 1 slice of buttered toast	46	9	medium
Amaretti biscuits (cookies)	21	1 biscuit	4	trace	low

Food	kC/ portion	Portion size	Carbs g	Fat g	Fibre
Amaretto liqueur	**80**	1 single measure	7	0	0
American hard gums	**135**	1 small tube	40	0	0
American muffin, plain	**169**	1 muffin	24	6	medium
American pancake	**60**	1 pancake	8	2	low
Anchovies, canned	**12**	1 fillet	0	1	0
Anchovies, fresh, grilled (broiled)	**98**	1 fish	0	4	0
Anchovy essence (extract)	**7**	1 tsp	0	trace	0
Anchovy paste	**20**	1 tbsp	trace	1	0
Angel cake	**77**	1 slice	12	trace	low
Angel delight, all flavours, made with semi-skimmed milk	**115** (avge)	1 serving	16	4	0
Angel delight, all flavours, made with skimmed milk	**105** (avge)	1 serving	16	2	0
Angel delight, sugar-free, all flavours, made with semi-skimmed milk	**115** (avge)	1 serving	13	5	0
Angel delight, sugar-free, all flavours, made with skimmed milk	**105** (avge)	1 serving	13	4	0
Angel hair (pasta strands), dried, boiled	**239**	1 serving	51	2	medium

Food	kCl/portion	Portion size	Carbs g	Fat g	Fibre
Angel hair, fresh, boiled	301	1 serving	57	2	medium
Angels on horseback	37	1 oyster plus ½ rasher (slice) of bacon	trace	3	0
Anis	55	1 single measure	trace	0	0
Aniseed balls	81	1 small tube	87	trace	0
Antipasti, mixed	244	1 serving	11	13	high
Anzac biscuits (cookies)	98	1 biscuit	4	5	low
Apple	47	1 fruit, unpeeled	12	trace	high
Apple, cooking (tart)	35	1 large fruit, peeled	9	trace	medium
Apple, cooking, baked, sweetened	140	1 large fruit	12	trace	high
Apple, dried rings	13	1 ring	3	trace	high
Apple, dried rings, stewed	66	3 heaped tbsp	13	trace	high
Apple, dried rings, stewed with sugar	106	3 heaped tbsp	17	trace	high
Apple, stewed	33	3 heaped tbsp	8	trace	medium
Apple, stewed with sugar	74	3 heaped tbsp	19	trace	medium
Apple, toffee	251	1 medium fruit	66	trace	high
Apple amber	340	1 serving	14	2	medium
Apple and blackcurrant juice drink	74	1 tumbler	16	trace	0
Apple and mango juice drink	67	1 tumbler	13	trace	0

Food	kC/ portion	Portion size	Carbs g	Fat g	Fibre
Apple betty	260	1 serving	39	10	medium
Apple cake	252	1 slice	32	10	medium
Apple charlotte	263	1 serving	41	9	medium
Apple chutney	30	1 tbsp	3	trace	low
Apple croissant	144	1 croissant	21	5	medium
Apple crumble	297	1 serving	51	10	medium
Apple danish pastry	298	1 pastry	51	18	medium
Apple drink, sparkling	78	1 tumbler	19	trace	0
Apple drink, sparkling, low-calorie	9	1 tumbler	2	trace	0
Apple dumpling	287	1 dumpling	54	8	high
Apple fritter	136	1 fritter	26	5	medium
Apple jelly (clear conserve)	67	1 tbsp	17	0	low
Apple juice, pure	76	1 tumbler	10	trace	low
Apple juice drink, diluted	88	1 tumbler	21	trace	0
Apple pie	290	1 slice	39	14	medium
Apple sauce	25	1 tbsp	2	trace	medium
Apple snow	97	1 serving	19	1	medium
Apple strudel	194	1 slice	29	8	medium
Apple tango	78	1 tumbler	19	trace	0
Apple tango, light	9	1 tumbler	2	trace	0
Apple turnover	284	1 turnover	31	16	medium

Food	kCl/portion	Portion size	Carbs g	Fat g	Fibre
Apricot	17	1 fruit	4	trace	medium
Apricot and almond danish pastry	270	1 pastry	38	12	medium
Apricot bites, dry	70	25 g/1 oz/½ cup	13	1	high
Apricot bites, with semi-skimmed milk	169	3 heaped tbsp	27	2	high
Apricot bites, with skimmed milk	153	3 heaped tbsp	27	3	high
Apricot brandy	56	1 single measure	7	0	0
Apricot jam (conserve)	39	1 tbsp	10	0	0
Apricot juice	78	1 tumbler	20	trace	0
Apricot nectar	112	1 tumbler	32	trace	0
Apricot sorbet	57	1 scoop	19	trace	low
Apricots, canned in natural juice	34	3 heaped tbsp	8	trace	medium
Apricots, canned in syrup	63	3 heaped tbsp	16	trace	medium
Apricots, dried	15	1 fruit	3	trace	high
Apricots, dried, stewed	85	3 heaped tbsp	22	trace	high
Apricots, dried, stewed with sugar	113	3 heaped tbsp	29	trace	high
Apricots, stewed	31	3 heaped tbsp	7	trace	medium
Apricots, stewed with sugar	61	3 heaped tbsp	15	trace	medium

Food	kC/ portion	Portion size	Carbs g	Fat g	Fibre
Arbroath smokies, grilled (broiled), with butter	239	1 fish	0	10	0
Archers peach liqueur	65	1 single measure	8	0	0
Arctic roll	100	1 slice	16	3	low
Arrowroot biscuits (cookies), thin	35	1 biscuit	7	2	low
Artichoke, globe, boiled	70	1 artichoke	3	0	medium
Artichoke, with melted butter	181	1 artichoke	3	13	medium
Artichoke hearts, canned, drained	8	1 heart	1	trace	medium
Artichoke vinaigrette	211	1 artichoke	3	22	medium
Artichokes, Jerusalem, boiled	41	3 heaped tbsp	11	0	high
Asparagus, canned, drained	24	½ medium can	1	trace	medium
Asparagus, roasted in olive oil	161	6 thick or 10 thin spears	1	16	medium
Asparagus, steamed or boiled	26	6 thick or 10 thin spears	2	2	medium
Asparagus, with melted butter	137	6 thick or 10 thin spears	1	13	medium
Asparagus quiche	320	1 slice	18	22	medium
Asparagus soup, cream of, canned	132	2 ladlefuls	10	10	low

Food	kCl/ portion	Portion size	Carbs g	Fat g	Fibre
Asparagus soup, cream of, instant	143	1 mug	20	6	low
Asparagus soup, home-made	167	2 ladlefuls	7	14	high
Aubergine (eggplant), fried (sautéed) in oil	302	¼ aubergine	3	32	medium
Aubergine, steamed or boiled	28	¼ aubergine	3	trace	medium
Aubergine, stuffed with meat	510	½ aubergine	28	24	medium
Aubergine, stuffed with savoury rice	523	½ aubergine	26	14	high
Aubergine dip	20	2 tbsp	4	1	medium
Austrian coffee cake	488	1 slice	41	32	low
Austrian smoked cheese	60	¼ barrel (25 g/1 oz)	trace	3	0
Avgolemono soup	74	2 ladlefuls	5	2	low
Avocado	286	1 medium fruit	3	29	medium
Avocado, baked, with tomato and cheese	196	½ avocado	4	18	medium
Avocado, with prawns (shrimp) in cocktail sauce	356	½ avocado	2	32	medium
Avocado vinaigrette	240	½ avocado	1	25	medium

Food	kC/ portion	Portion size	Carbs g	Fat g	Fibre
Babybel cheese	53	1 cheese	0	4	0
Bacardi	50	1 single measure	trace	trace	0
Bacardi and coke	94	1 single measure plus 1 mixer	6	0	0
Bacardi and diet coke	56	1 single measure plus 1 mixer	trace	0	0
Baclava	322	1 pastry	40	17	medium
Bacon, back, lean, fried (sautéed)	133	1 rasher (slice)	0	16	0
Bacon, back, lean, grilled (broiled)	117	1 rasher	0	8	0
Bacon, joint, boiled	325	2 thick slices	0	27	0
Bacon, joint, honey-roasted	346	2 thick slices	4	27	0
Bacon, streaky, fried	149	1 rasher	0	13	0
Bacon, streaky, grilled	127	1 rasher	0	11	0
Bacon and egg quiche	387	1 slice	17	31	low
Bacon and egg mcmuffin	346	1 muffin	26	18	medium
Bacon and mushroom pizza, deep-pan	340	1 slice	35	16	medium
Bacon and mushroom pizza, thin-crust	290	1 slice	25	15	medium
Bacon cheeseburger	400	1 burger	27	22	low

Food	kCl/ portion	Portion size	Carbs g	Fat g	Fibre
Bacon sandwiches	**538**	1 round	34	32	medium
Bagel	**228**	1 bagel	44	3	medium
Bagna cauda	**499**	1 individual pot	0	52	0
Baguette	**364**	1 small	75	2	medium
Bailey's irish cream	**80**	1 single measure	6	4	0
Baked alaska	**339**	1 serving	62	8	low
Baked beans	**168**	1 small can	31	1	high
Baked beans, barbecued	164	1 small can	30	1	high
Baked beans, on toast	323	1 small can plus 1 slice of toast	49	10	high
Baked beans, reduced-sugar and reduced-salt	146	1 small can	25	1	high
Baked beans, reduced-sugar and reduced-salt, on toast	301	1 small can plus 1 slice of toast	43	10	high
Baked beans, with bacon	182	1 small can plus 2 rashers (slices) of bacon	26	3	high
Baked beans, with burgers, canned	206	1 small can	26	6	high
Baked beans, with sausages, canned	220	1 small can	26	9	high
Baked beans, with vegetarian sausages, canned	240	1 small can	63	trace	high

Food	kC/ portion	Portion size	Carbs g	Fat g	Fibre
Bakewell slice	156	1 slice	22	7	medium
Bakewell tart	297	1 slice	37	15	medium
Balsamic vinegar	2	1 tsp	1	0	0
Bamboo shoots	6	2 tbsp	trace	trace	medium
Banana	95	1 medium fruit	23	trace	medium
Banana, dried slices	78	1 small handful	9	5	medium
Banana bread	246	1 slice	45	7	medium
Banana custard	50	5 tbsp	8	1	0
Banana flambé	250	1 banana	28	8	medium
Banana fritter	175	1 fritter	33	5	medium
Banana milkshake, fresh, made with semi-skimmed milk	163	1 tumbler	31	3	medium
Banana milkshake, fresh, made with skimmed milk	144	1 tumbler	31	trace	medium
Banana sandwiches	399	1 round	57	17	medium
Banana split	481	1 serving	77	16	medium
Bananabix, dry	92	25 g/1 oz/½ cup	18	trace	high
Bananabix, with semi-skimmed milk	207	3 heaped tbsp	35	4	high
Bananabix, with skimmed milk	191	3 heaped tbsp	35	3	high

Food	kC/ portion	Portion size	Carbs g	Fat g	Fibre
Bangers and mash	462	2 sausages plus 4 spoonfuls of mash	43	20	medium
Banoffee pie	574	1 slice	68	23	medium
Barbecue sauce	11	1 tbsp	1	trace	0
Barbecued baked beans	164	1 small can	30	1	high
Barbecued chicken	287	1 chicken portion	1	10	0
Barbecued pork chop	210	1 chop	1	9	0
Barbecued spare ribs	288	2 ribs	2	16	0
Barley sugar	96	1 stick	24	0	0
Barley water, all flavours	40 (avge)	1 tumbler	9	trace	0
Barley water, all flavours, no added sugar	6 (avge)	1 tumbler	1	trace	0
Barley wine	120	1 small bottle	11	trace	0
Bass, fried (sautéed), in seasoned flour	261	1 piece of fillet	5	12	low
Bass, grilled (broiled)	142	1 piece of fillet	0	2	0
Bass, poached	141	1 piece of fillet	0	2	0
Bass, stuffed, baked	182	1 serving	1	4	low
Bath bun	263	1 bun	45	15	medium
Bath olivers	50	1 biscuit (cookie)	8	2	low
Battenburg cake	370	1 slice	50	17	medium

Food	kC/ portion	Portion size	Carbs g	Fat g	Fibre
Bavarian smoked cheese	60	¼ barrel (25 g/1 oz)	trace	3	0
Bavarois, all flavours	308 (avge)	1 serving	17	23	0
Bean and cheese enchiladas	547	2 enchiladas	82	14	high
Bean salad	120	3 heaped tbsp	12	5	high
Beanburger, spicy	112	1 burger	4	6	medium
Beans See *individual varieties, e.g.* Runner beans					
Beansprouts	8	1 good handful	1	trace	high
Béarnaise sauce	275	5 tbsp	7	27	low
Béchamel sauce, made with semi-skimmed milk	96	5 tbsp	8	6	low
Beef, boiled	326	2 thick slices	0	24	0
Beef, corned	54	1 slice	0	3	0
Beef, grillsteak, grilled (broiled)	185	1 steak	8	12	low
Beef, minced (ground), in gravy, canned	230	½ large can	14	11	0
Beef, minced, lean, stewed	229	1 serving	0	15	0
Beef, roast, lean	225	4 thin slices	0	19	0
Beef, steak See Steak					
Beef, stewed in gravy	335	1 serving	0	16	0

Food	kCl/portion	Portion size	Carbs g	Fat g	Fibre
Beef, stewed in gravy, canned	254	½ large can	8	10	0
Beef and cheese enchiladas	644	2 enchiladas	60	36	low
Beef and tomato soup, canned	88	2 ladlefuls	10	2	low
Beef and tomato soup, instant	72	1 mug	15	1	0
Beef and vegetable stir-fry	433	1 serving	71	5	high
Beef broth, canned	76	2 ladlefuls	13	1	low
Beef carbonnade (in beer)	384	1 serving	15	21	low
Beef casserole	360	1 serving	13	21	medium
Beef chop suey	297	1 serving	34	6	medium
Beef chow mein	408	1 serving	43	18	high
Beef consommé, canned	14	2 ladlefuls	1	trace	0
Beef consommé, jellied	21	2 ladlefuls	1	trace	0
Beef curry, home-made	905	1 serving	10	77	medium
Beef curry, home-made, with rice	1153	1 serving	66	79	medium
Beef curry, retail	411	1 serving	19	18	medium
Beef curry, retail, with rice	657	1 serving	82	19	medium
Beef fajitas	528	2 fajitas	79	8	medium
Beef goulash	406	1 serving	16	22	medium
Beef in oyster sauce	204	1 serving	10	8	low
Beef kheema	826	1 serving	1	75	low

Food	kCl/portion	Portion size	Carbs g	Fat g	Fibre
Beef koftas	**441**	1 serving	4	35	low
Beef olives	**494**	2 olives	20	18	low
Beef pie	**460**	1 individual pie	32	28	low
Beef pot roast, with vegetables	**420**	1 serving	14	15	medium
Beef risotto	**452**	1 serving	54	29	low
Beef satay	**222**	1 skewer	6	11	low
Beef sausages, thick, fried (sautéed)	**108**	1 sausage	6	7	low
Beef sausages, thick, grilled (broiled)	**106**	1 sausage	6	7	low
Beef sausages, thin, fried	**54**	1 sausage	4	4	low
Beef sausages, thin, grilled	**53**	1 sausage	4	4	low
Beef spread	**35**	1 tbsp	2	3	low
Beef steak pudding	**684**	1 serving	57	37	medium
Beef stew	**360**	1 serving	13	21	medium
Beef stroganoff	**361**	1 serving	8	25	medium
Beef teriyaki	**128**	1 serving	2	4	low
Beef wellington	**527**	1 serving	23	33	low
Beef with mushrooms, chinese	**320**	1 serving	44	6	low
Beef with pineapple, chinese	**337**	1 serving	47	6	low
See *also* Boeuf					

Food	kCl/portion	Portion size	Carbs g	Fat g	Fibre
Beefburger, fried (sautéed)	**125**	1 burger	trace	11	0
Beefburger, grilled (broiled)	**122**	1 burge	trace	11	0
Beefburger, in a bun, quarterpounder	**321**	1 burger in a bun	27	15	medium
Beefburger, in a bun, small	**246**	1 burger in a bun	23	13	medium
Beer, bitter	**96**	1 small	7	trace	0
Beer, extra-strength	**216**	1 small	18	trace	0
Beer, pale ale	**96**	1 small	6	trace	0
Beerwurst	**55**	1 slice	trace	4	0
Beetroot (red beet)	**36**	1 medium	7	trace	medium
Beetroot, boiled	**46**	1 medium	9	trace	medium
Beetroot, pickled	**28**	5 slices	6	trace	medium
Bel paese cheese	**87**	1 small wedge	trace	7	0
Belgian bun	**192**	1 bun	30	5	low
Belgian endive See Chicory					
Belgian ham, dry-cured	**21**	1 slice	0	1	0
Bell pepper See Pepper					
Benedictine	**90**	1 single measure	6	0	0
Big bar ace	**204**	1 standard bar	25	10	low
Big breakfast	**591**	1 meal	40	36	high
Big fish sandwich	**720**	1 bun	59	43	high

Food	kC/ portion	Portion size	Carbs g	Fat g	Fibre
Big mac	493	1 burger	44	23	high
Bigarde sauce	123	5 tbsp	10	4	low
Biscotti	39	1 biscuit (cookie)	6	1	low
Biscuits (cookies), chocolate, full-coated	131	1 biscuit	17	7	low
Biscuits, chocolate, half-coated	84	1 biscuit	11	4	low
Biscuits, cream-filled	77	1 biscuit	10	4	low
Biscuits, semi-sweet	46	1 biscuit	7	2	low
Biscuits, short, sweet	47	1 biscuit	6	2	low
Biscuits, wafer, cream-filled	39	1 biscuit	5	3	low
See also individual names, e.g. Hobnob					
Bitter lemon, sparkling	68	1 tumbler	16	0	0
Bitter orange, sparkling	68	1 tumbler	16	0	0
Black bean sauce	22	1 tbsp	3	trace	low
Black beans, dried, soaked and cooked	103	3 heaped tbsp	18	trace	high
Black cherries, canned in syrup	71	3 heaped tbsp	18	trace	low
Black cherry cheesecake	242	1 slice	33	11	low
Black cherry jam (conserve)	39	1 tbsp	10	0	0
Black cherry jam, reduced-sugar	6	1 tbsp	5	0	0
Black forest gateau	432	1 slice	65	18	low

B

Food	kC/ portion	Portion size	Carbs g	Fat g	Fibre
Black forest ham	29	1 thin slice	trace	2	0
Black gram, boiled	45	1 serving	7	trace	low
Black jack chew sweets (candies)	15	1 sweet	3	trace	0
Black pudding, fried (sautéed)	305	2 thick slices	15	22	low
Black velvet	168	1 cocktail	5	trace	0
Blackberries	25	3 heaped tbsp	5	trace	high
Blackberries, stewed	21	3 heaped tbsp	4	trace	medium
Blackberries, stewed with sugar	56	3 heaped tbsp	14	trace	medium
Blackberry and apple crumble	297	1 serving	51	10	medium
Blackberry and apple pie	281	1 slice	11	39	medium
Blackberry jam (conserve)	39	1 tbspe	10	0	0
Blackcurrant and apple pie	378	1 slice	56	16	medium
Blackcurrant and apple squash, diluted	58	1 tumbler	15	0	0
Blackcurrant cheesecake	260	1 slice	38	12	low
Blackcurrant cordial, diluted	103	1 tumbler	27	0	0
Blackcurrant crumble	298	1 serving	51	10	medium
Blackcurrant jam (conserve)	39	1 tbsp	10	0	0
Blackcurrant jam, reduced-sugar	6	1 tbsp	0	0	
Blackcurrant juice drink	120	1 tumbler	32	trace	0

Food	kCal/portion	Portion size	Carbs g	Fat g	Fibre
Blackcurrant pastilles	**131**	1 small tube	32	0	0
Blackcurrant pie	**282**	1 slice	34	13	medium
Blackcurrant sorbet	**65**	1 scoop	17	trace	0
Blackcurrants	**28**	3 heaped tbsp	7	trace	high
Blackcurrants, canned in natural juice	**31**	3 heaped tbsp	8	trace	medium
Blackcurrants, canned in syrup	**72**	3 heaped tbsp	18	trace	medium
Blackcurrants, stewed with sugar	**58**	3 heaped tbsp	15	trace	medium
Black-eyed beans, dried, soaked and cooked	**116**	3 heaped tbsp	20	1	high
Blancmange	**165**	1 serving	23	6	low
Blewits, fried (sautéed)	**78**	2 tbsp	trace	8	low
Blewits, stewed	**6**	2 tbsp	trace	trace	low
Blinis	**60**	1 pancake	8	2	low
Blintzes	**86**	1 pancake	11	1	low
Bloater, grilled (broiled)	**298**	1 fish	0	19	0
Bloater paste	**5**	1 tsp	1	trace	low
Bloody mary	**69**	1 cocktail	3	trace	low
Bloomer loaf	**70**	1 medium slice	15	1	low
BLT	**650**	1 round	34	35	medium
Blue brie cheese	**106**	1 small wedge	trace	10	0

Food	kCl/ portion	Portion size	Carbs g	Fat g	Fibre
Blue chartreuse	**78**	1 single measure	7	0	0
Blue cheese dip	**145**	1 small pot	trace	12	0
Blue cheese dressing	**77**	1 tbsp	1	8	0
Blue cheese dressing, low-calorie	**16**	1 tbsp	2	1	0
Blue riband chocolate wafer	**108**	1 standard bar	13	6	low
Blue stilton cheese	**103**	1 small wedge	trace	9	0
Blueberries	**56**	3 heaped tbsp	14	trace	medium
Blueberries, canned in syrup	**88**	3 heaped tbsp	22	trace	medium
Blueberries, dried	**44**	1 small handful	12	trace	high
Blueberries, stewed	**51**	3 heaped tbsp	12	trace	medium
Blueberries, stewed with sugar	**81**	3 heaped tbsp	22	trace	medium
Blueberry buster muffin	**408**	1 muffin	47	21	medium
Blueberry muffin	**294**	1 large muffin	38	14	medium
Blueberry pie	**290**	1 slice	39	14	medium
Bluefish, grilled (broiled)	**186**	1 fillet	0	6	0
Boasters biscuits (cookies), all flavours	**90** (avge)	1 biscuit	20	5	low
Bockwurst	**199**	1 sausage	trace	18	0
Boeuf bourguignon	**450**	1 serving	7	33	low
Boeuf en daube	**351**	1 serving	14	13	medium
See *also* Beef					

Food	kCl/portion	Portion size	Carbs g	Fat g	Fibre
Boiled beef with carrots and dumplings	474	1 serving	29	26	medium
Boiled sweets (candies)	15	1 sweet	5	trace	0
Bologna sausage	57	1 slice	trace	5	0
Bolognese sauce	217	1 serving	5	17	low
Bolony sausage	57	1 slice	trace	5	0
Bombay mix snack	75	1 small handful	2	5	high
Bon bel cheese	78	1 small wedge	0	6	0
Bon-bons	28	1 sweet (candy)	6	trace	0
Bonito, grilled (broiled)	195	1 piece of fillet	0	7	0
Boost chocolate bar	295	1 standard bar	34	16	low
Bordelaise sauce	133	5 tbsp	2	4	0
Borlotti beans, canned, drained	112	3 heaped tbsp	8	trace	high
Borlotti beans, dried, soaked and cooked	116	3 heaped tbsp	18	1	high
Bortsch	25	2 ladlefuls	1	1	high
Bortsch, jellied	50	2 ladlefuls	1	1	high
Boston baked beans	133	1 serving	26	1	high
Boudoir biscuits (lady fingers)	40	1 finger	6	1	low
Bouillabaise	159	2 ladlefuls	21	2	medium
Bouillabaise with rouille	310	2 ladlefuls	23	17	medium

Food	kC/ portion	Portion size	Carbs g	Fat g	Fibre
Bounty bar, milk chocolate	289	1 standard bar	32	15	low
Bounty bar, plain (semi-sweet) chocolate	276	1 standard bar	33	15	low
Bounty, ice cream bar	299	1 standard bar	24	21	low
Bourbon	60	1 single measure	trace	0	0
Bourbon biscuits (cookies)	63	1 biscuit	9	3	low
Bournville chocolate	250	1 standard bar	30	13	0
Bournvita, made with semi-skimmed milk	145	1 mug	19	4	low
Bournvita, made with skimmed milk	137	1 mug	20	2	low
Boursin cheese, all flavours	77 (avge)	1 heaped tbsp	1	7	0
Boursin, light, all flavours	28 (avge)	1 heaped tbsp	1	2	0
Bovril	3	1 tsp	trace	trace	0
Bran, oat	51	1 tbsp	9	1	high
Bran, wheat	31	1 tbsp	4	1	high
Bran muffin	163	1 muffin	24	6	high
Brandy	55	1 single measure	trace	0	0
Brandy alexander	270	1 cocktail	18	0	
Brandy butter	73	1 tbsp	8	4	0

Food	kC/ portion	Portion size	Carbs g	Fat g	Fibre
Brandy sauce, made with semi-skimmed milk	**50**	5 tbsp	5	2	low
Brandy sauce, made with skimmed milk	**47**	5 tbsp	5	trace	low
Brandy snaps	**57**	1 snap	10	2	low
Brandy sour	**57**	1 cocktail	trace	trace	0
Branflakes, dry	**80**	25 g/1 oz/½ cup	16	1	high
Branflakes, with semi skimmed milk-	**185**	5 heaped tbsp	33	3	high
Branflakes, with skimmed milk	**169**	5 heaped tbsp	33	1	high
Branflakes, with sultanas (golden raisins), dry	**80**	25 g/1 oz/½ cup	16	trace	high
Branflakes, with sultanas, with skimmed milk	**169**	5 heaped tbsp	33	1	high
Branflakes, with sultanas, with semi-skimmed milk	**185**	5 heaped tbsp	33	3	high
Bratwurst, fried (sautéed)	**256**	1 sausage	2	22	0
Brazil nut, shelled	**23**	1 nut	trace	3	high
Brazil nut toffee	**39**	1 toffee	5	2	low
Brazils, chocolate	**49**	1 sweet (candy)	3	4	high
Bread, brown, medium-sliced	**78**	1 slice	16	1	medium
Bread, brown, medium-sliced, toasted	**80**	1 slice	16	1	medium

Food	kCl/ portion	Portion size	Carbs g	Fat g	Fibre
Bread, brown, thick-sliced	109	1 slice	22	1	medium
Bread, brown, thin-sliced	65	1 slice	13	1	medium
Bread, granary, medium-sliced	94	1 slice	18	1	medium
Bread, granary, medium-sliced, toasted	96	1 slice	18	1	medium
Bread, granary, thick-sliced	117	1 slice	23	2	medium
Bread, softgrain medium-sliced	76	1 slice	15	1	medium
Bread, softgrain, medium-sliced, toasted	85	1 slice	18	1	medium
Bread, softgrain, thick-sliced	106	1 slice	21	1	medium
Bread, white, medium-sliced	78	1 slice	17	trace	low
Bread, white, medium-sliced, toasted	81	1 slice	18	trace	low
Bread, white, thick-sliced	108	1 slice	23	trace	low
Bread, white, thin-sliced	65	1 slice	14	trace	low
Bread, wholemeal, medium-sliced	77	1 slice	15	1	high
Bread, wholemeal, medium-sliced, toasted	79	1 slice	15	1	high
Bread, wholemeal, thick-sliced	107	1 slice	21	1	high
Bread, wholemeal, thin-sliced	64	1 slice	12	1	high
Bread, with butter	152 (avge)	1 medium slice	17	9	low

Food	kC/ portion	Portion size	Carbs g	Fat g	Fibre
Bread, with low-fat spread	117 (avge)	1 medium slice	17	4	low
Bread pudding	297	1 serving	50	10	medium
Bread and butter pudding	280	1 serving	31	13	low
Bread roll, baton	182	1 roll	38	1	medium
Bread roll, brown	134	1 roll	26	2	medium
Bread roll, crusty	140	1 roll	29	2	low
Bread roll, finger	107	1 roll	21	2	low
Bread roll, granary	117	1 roll	23	1	medium
Bread roll, hamburger bun	132	1 bun	24	2	low
Bread roll, soft white bap	134	1 roll	26	2	low
Bread roll, starch–reduced	50	1 roll	10	trace	low
Bread roll, wholemeal	120	1 roll	24	1	high
Bread roll, with butter	214 (avge)	1 roll	29	9	low
Bread roll, with low-fat spread	179 (avge)	1 roll	29	5	low
Bread sauce, made with semi-skimmed milk	14	1 tbsp	2	trace	low
Bread sauce, made with skimmed milk	12	1 tbsp	2	trace	low
Breadfruit	396	1 medium fruit	104	trace	high

Food	kCl/portion	Portion size	Carbs g	Fat g	Fibre
Breadfruit, canned, drained	66	3 heaped tbsp	16	trace	medium
Breadsticks	20	1 stick	3	trace	low
Breakaway chocolate bar, caramac	125	1 standard bar	13	7	low
Breakaway, milk	114	1 standard bar	14	6	low
Breakfast compôte, canned	73	3 heaped tbsp	17	trace	high
Bream, fried (sautéed) in seasoned flour	261	1 piece of fillet	5	12	low
Bream, grilled (broiled)	142	1 piece of fillet	0	2	0
Bream, poached	141	1 piece of fillet	0	2	0
Bresaola	15	1 thin slice	trace	trace	0
Bresse bleu cheese	106	1 small wedge	trace	10	0
Brie cheese	80	1 small wedge	trace	7	0
Brill, fried (sautéed) in egg and breadcrumbs	342	1 piece of fillet	13	20	low
Brill, grilled (broiled)	126	1 piece of fillet	0	3	0
Brill, poached	125	1 piece of fillet	0	2	0
Brioche	140	1 brioche	22	4	low
Brisket of beef, boiled	326	2 thick slices	0	24	0
Broad (fava) beans, boiled	48	3 heaped tbsp	6	1	high
Broad beans, canned, drained	77	3 heaped tbsp	13	trace	high
Broad beans, frozen, cooked	81	3 heaped tbsp	12	1	high

Food	kC/ portion	Portion size	Carbs g	Fat g	Fibre
Broccoli, steamed or boiled	33	4 medium florets	2	1	medium
Broccoli and cauliflower soup, instant	59	1 mug	8	2	low
Broccoli and cauliflower soup, packet	110	2 ladlefuls	15	5	medium
Broccoli and cheese quiche	320	1 slice	18	22	low
Broccoli and cheese soup, canned	132	2 ladlefuls	9	7	medium
Broccoli and cheese soup, home-made	169	2 ladlefuls	21	6	high
Broccoli in cheese sauce, made with semi-skimmed milk	167	1 serving	9	11	medium
Broccoli in cheese sauce, made with skimmed milk	157	1 serving	9	9	medium
Broccoli soup	118	2 ladlefuls	21	2	high
Brown ale	84	1 small	9	trace	0
Brown betty	260	1 serving	39	10	medium
Brown sauce	15	1 tbsp	4	0	low
Brownie, chocolate	368	1 brownie	63	11	medium
Brunswick stew	444	1 serving	46	12	high
Brussels sprouts, steamed or boiled	35	3 heaped tbsp	3	1	high

Food	kC/ portion	Portion size	Carbs g	Fat g	Fibre
Brussels sprouts, with chestnuts	**176**	3 heaped tbsp	20	43	high
Bubble and squeak	**240**	1 serving	7	18	high
Bucatini (long macaroni), dried, boiled	**239**	1 serving	51	2	medium
Bucatini, fresh, boiled	**301**	1 serving	57	2	medium
Buck rarebit	**312**	1 slice	22	19	low
Buckling, smoked	**520**	1 fish	0	44	0
Buckwheat noodles, boiled	**228**	1 serving	48	trace	low
Buckwheat pancakes	**45**	1 pancake	6	2	low
Bulgar (cracked wheat), cooked	**177**	3 heaped tbsp	29	4	medium
Buns *See individual flavours, e.g. Currant bun*					
Burger bun	**132**	1 bun	24	2	low
Burgers *See individual varieties, e.g. Hamburger*					
Burritos, with beans and cheese	**377**	2 burritos	55	12	medium
Burritos, with beef, beans and cheese	**331**	2 burritos	40	13	medium
Butter	**184**	25 g/1 oz/2 tbsp	trace	20	0
Butter	**74**	1 small knob	trace	8	0
Butter (lima) beans, canned, drained	**77**	3 heaped tbsp	13	trace	high

Food	kC/ portion	Portion size	Carbs g	Fat g	Fibre
Butter beans, dried, soaked and cooked	103	3 heaped tbsp	18	1	high
Butter pecan ice cream	91	1 scoop	12	4	low
Butter puffs	54	1 biscuit	6	3	low
Butter sauce	112	5 tbsp	8	8	low
Butter shortcake biscuits (cookies)	50	1 biscuit	7	2	low
Butter/vegetable fat spread	165	25 g/1 oz/2 tbsp	trace	18	0
Butter/vegetable fat spread	66	1 small knob	trace	7	0
Buttercream icing (frosting)	40	1 tbsp	9	3	0
Butterfly cakes	245	1 individual cake	26	15	low
Butterfly prawns (jumbo shrimp), fried (sautéed), in breadcrumbs	405	6 prawns	35	23	low
Buttermilk	60	150 ml/¼ pt/⅔ cup	8	trace	0
Butternut squash, steamed or boiled	9	½ medium squash	2	trace	low
Butterscotch	24	1 piece	5	trace	0
Butterscotch sauce	145	2 tbsp	32	2	low
Butterscotch tart	531	1 slice	57	23	low

Food	kC/ portion	Portion size	Carbs g	Fat g	Fibre

Food	kC/ portion	Portion size	Carbs g	Fat g	Fibre
Cabbage, green, steamed or boiled	**16**	3 heaped tbsp	2	trace	medium
Cabbage, red/white, pickled	**3**	1 tbsp	trace	0	medium
Cabbage, red/white, raw	**27**	3 heaped tbsp	5	trace	medium
Cabbage leaves, stuffed	**221**	2 leaves	19	9	high
Cabinet pudding	**233**	1 serving	36	2	medium
Caerphilly cheese	**94**	1 small wedge	trace	8	0
Caesar salad	**207**	1 serving	6	13	medium
Café noir biscuits (cookies)	**39**	1 biscuit	8	trace	low
Caffé latte	**133**	1 medium cup	10	8	0
Cajun chicken	**366**	1 serving	33	9	0
Cake, chocolate	**384**	1 slice	58	14	low
Cake, light fruit	**354**	1 slice	58	13	medium
Cake, plain	**393**	1 slice	58	17	low
Cake, rich fruit	**341**	1 slice	60	11	medium
See also Sponge cake and individual flavours, e.g. Coffee cake					
Calabrese, steamed or boiled	**33**	4 medium florets	2	1	medium
Calamari rings, fried (sautéed), in batter	**235**	1 serving	19	12	low
Calippo ice lolly, any flavour	**105**	1 lolly	26	trace	0

Food	kC/portion	Portion size	Carbs g	Fat g	Fibre
Calvados	**55**	1 single measure	trace	0	0
Calves' liver, braised	**165**	3 thin slices	3	7	low
Calves' liver, fried (sautéed), in seasoned flour	**254**	3 thin slices	7	13	0
Calypso coffee	**218**	1 wine glass	7	14	0
Calzone	**470**	1 individual pie	50	24	medium
Cambozola cheese	**106**	1 small wedge	trace	10	0
Camembert cheese	**74**	1 small wedge	trace	6	0
Camp coffee, made with semi-skimmed milk	**125**	1 mug	15	4	0
Camp coffee, made with skimmed milk	**93**	1 mug	15	trace	0
Candied fruits See Glacé fruits					
Candied peel See Mixed peel					
Candy See *individual varieties, e.g.* Chocolate brazils, Lemon drops					
Candy floss	**100**	1 stick	26	0	0
Cannellini beans, canned, drained	**101**	3 heaped tbsp	22	1	high
Cannellini beans, dried, soaked and cooked	**103**	3 heaped tbsp	17	trace	high
Cannelloni, filled with meat	**298**	2 tubes	24	17	medium

Food	kCl portion	Portion size	Carbs g	Fat g	Fibre
Cannelloni, filled with spinach and ricotta	250	2 tubes	17	16	medium
Cantal cheese	101	1 small wedge	trace	8	0
Canteloupe melon	57	½ melon	13	trace	medium
Cape gooseberries	3	1 fruit	trace	trace	low
Cappellini (pasta strands), dried, boiled	239	1 serving	51	2	medium
Cappellini, fresh, boiled	301	1 serving	57	2	medium
Caper sauce, made with semi-skimmed milk	103	5 tbsp	10	6	low
Caper sauce, made with skimmed milk	93	5 tbsp	10	5	low
Capercaillie, roast	173	¼ bird	0	5	0
Capers, pickled	7	1 tbsp	2	0	low
Capon, roast, with skin	216	3 medium slices	0	14	0
Capon, roast, without skin	148	3 medium slices	0	5	0
Caponata	85	1 slice	15	1	medium
Cappelletti (stuffed pasta), dried, all stuffings	291 (avge)	1 serving	45	6	medium
Cappelletti, fresh, all stuffings	229 (avge)	1 serving	40	4	medium
Cappuccino	101	1 medium cup	7	6	0
Capsicum See Pepper					

Food	kC/ portion	Portion size	Carbs g	Fat g	Fibre
Caramac chocolate bar	170	1 standard bar	16	11	0
Caramel ice cream	89	1 scoop	12	4	low
Caramel shortcake	171	1 slice	20	9	low
Caramel toffees	29	1 toffee	6	1	0
Caramel wafers	113	1 standard bar	17	5	low
Carbonara pasta sauce	163	¼ jar	5	20	0
Carob bar	470	1 standard bar	49	27	high
Carpaccio of beef	61	2 thin slices	0	2	0
Carrot	35	1 large carrot	8	trace	medium
Carrot and orange soup	78	2 ladlefuls	12	3	medium
Carrot cake	260	1 slice	47	7	medium
Carrot juice	24	1 small glass	6	trace	0
Carrots, honey-glazed	39	3 heaped tbsp	9	trace	medium
Carrots, steamed or boiled	24	3 heaped tbsp	5	trace	medium
Cashew nuts, fresh	143	25 g/1 oz/¼ cup	4	12	high
Cashew nuts, roasted	92	1 small handful	3	8	high
Cassata	227	1 serving	14	23	low
Cassava, baked	310	2 pieces	80	trace	high
Cassava, boiled	130	2 pieces	33	trace	high
Cassoulet	341	1 serving	38	13	high
Castle pudding	233	1 individual pudding	36	2	medium

Food	kC/ portion	Portion size	Carbs g	Fat g	Fibre
Catfish, fried (sautéed), in breadcrumbs	265	1 piece of fillet	9	15	low
Catfish, grilled (broiled)	217	1 piece of fillet	0	2	0
Catfish, steamed or poached	141	1 piece of fillet	0	2	0
Catsup See Ketchup					
Cauliflower	34	4 medium florets	3	1	medium
Cauliflower, in white sauce, made with semi-skimmed milk	124	3 heaped tbsp	10	7	medium
Cauliflower, in white sauce, made with skimmed milk	114	3 heaped tbsp	10	6	medium
Cauliflower, steamed or boiled	28	4 medium florets	2	1	medium
Cauliflower bhaji	150	1 bhaji	3	14	medium
Cauliflower cheese	157	1 serving	8	10	medium
Cauliflower soup	133	2 ladlefuls	16	5	medium
Caviar, red or black	40	1 tbsp	1	3	0
Celeriac (celery root)	20	¼ small head	3	trace	high
Celeriac, steamed or boiled	15	3 heaped tbsp	2	trace	high
Celery	2	1 stick	trace	trace	low
Celery, braised	8	3 heaped tbsp	1	trace	medium
Celery root See Celeriac					
Celery soup, cream of, canned	86	2 ladlefuls	7	6	low

Food	kC/ portion	Portion size	Carbs g	Fat g	Fibre
Celery soup, packet	50	2 ladlefuls	8	2	low
Celery soup, home-made	82	2 ladlefuls	11	2	medium
Cellophane noodles, boiled	251	1 serving	57	trace	low
Ceps mushrooms, stewed	6	2 tbsp	trace	trace	low
Cereal bars, chewy, all flavours	131 (avge)	1 bar	21	5	medium
Cereal bars, crunchy, all flavours	146 (avge)	1 bar	17	7	medium
Cervelat	77	1 slice	trace	7	0
Champagne	114	1 wine glass	2	0	0
Channa dahl	125	3 heaped tbsp	10	6	high
Chanterelle mushrooms, stewed	6	2 tbsp	trace	trace	low
Chantilly cream	72	1 tbsp	trace	8	0
Chapattis, made with fat	164	1 chapatti	24	6	medium
Chapattis, made without fat	101	1 chapatti	22	trace	medium
Charentais melon	57	½ melon	13	trace	medium
Chargrilled chicken sandwiches	401	1 round	29	20	medium
Chargrilled chicken breast	192	1 breast	0	4	0
Charlotte russe	307	1 serving	50	10	low
Chasseur sauce	36	5 tbsp	7	trace	0
Chaumes cheese	94	1 small wedge	trace	8	0

Food	kC/ portion	Portion size	Carbs g	Fat g	Fibre
Cheddar cheese	103	1 small wedge	trace	9	0
Cheddar cheese, low-fat	65	1 small wedge	trace	4	0
Cheddars	21	1 biscuit (cookie)	2	1	low
Cheerios, dry	92	25 g/1 oz/½ cup	18	1	medium
Cheerios, with semi-skimmed milk	204	5 heaped tbsp	36	3	medium
Cheerios, with skimmed milk	188	5 heaped tbsp	36	1	medium
Cheese, fresh, soft, full-fat	39	1 heaped tbsp	trace	4	0
Cheese, fresh, soft, low-fat	15	1 heaped tbsp	trace	trace	0
Cheese, fresh, soft, medium-fat	22	1 heaped tbsp	trace	2	0
Cheese, potted	267	1 individual pot	1	23	0
See also individual names, e.g. Cheddar					
Cheese and bean enchiladas	547	2 enchiladas	82	14	high
Cheese and beef enchiladas	644	2 enchiladas	60	36	low
Cheese and coleslaw sandwiches	440	1 round	36	28	medium
Cheese and ham sandwiches	432	1 round	34	27	medium
Cheese and onion quiche	396	1 slice	24	28	medium
Cheese and pickle sandwiches	407	1 round	34	26	medium
Cheese and pineapple chunks	25	1 stick	1	2	low
Cheese and tomato pizza, deep-pan	300	1 slice	30	14	medium

Food	kCl/ portion	Portion size	Carbs g	Fat g	Fibre
Cheese and tomato pizza, thin-crust	235	1 slice	25	12	medium
Cheese and tomato sandwiches	411	1 round	36	26	medium
Cheese fondue	492	1 serving	8	29	0
Cheese fondue, with French bread	762	1 serving plus 10 cubes of bread	62	31	low
Cheese footballs	13	1 football	1	1	low
Cheese melt biscuits (cookies)	21	1 biscuit	3	1	low
Cheese melt biscuits, mini	6	1 biscuit	1	trace	low
Cheese omelette	356	2 eggs	trace	30	0
Cheese on toast	223	1 slice	21	13	low
Cheese pudding	292	1 serving	24	14	low
Cheese sandwiches	398	1 round	34	26	medium
Cheese sauce, made with semi-skimmed milk	134	5 tbsp	7	10	low
Cheese sauce, made with skimmed milk	124	5 tbsp	7	8	low
Cheese scone (biscuit)	175	1 scone	21	9	low
Cheese scone, with butter	249	1 scone	21	17	low
Cheese scone, with low-fat spread	214	1 scone	21	13	low
Cheese slice, processed	65	1 slice	trace	5	0

Food	kC/ portion	Portion size	Carbs g	Fat g	Fibre
Cheese soufflé	**280**	1 serving	10	9	low
Cheese soup, canned	**126**	2 ladlefuls	8	8	low
Cheese soup, home-made	**94**	2 ladlefuls	11	3	low
Cheese spread	**41**	1 tbsp	1	3	0
Cheese spread, low-fat	**27**	1 tbsp	1	2	0
Cheese spread, flavoured	**35**	1 tbsp	1	3	low
Cheese straws	**28**	1 straw	2	trace	low
Cheeseburger	**299**	1 burger in a bun	33	11	medium
Cheesecake, plain, cooked	**490**	1 slice	30	27	low
Cheesecake, plain, set	**272**	1 slice	30	13	low
Cheesecake, with fruit topping	**302**	1 slice	41	13	low
See also individual flavours, e.g. Chocolate cheesecake					
Cheeselets	**147**	1 small bag	16	8	medium
Chelsea bun	**329**	1 bun	50	12	medium
Cherries	**20**	10 cherries	4	trace	low
Cherries, canned in natural juice	**51**	3 heaped tbsp	13	trace	low
Cherries, canned in syrup	**71**	3 heaped tbsp	18	trace	low
Cherries, glacé (candied)	**13**	1 cherry	4	trace	low
Cherries, in brandy/kirsch	**126**	3 heaped tbsp	18	trace	low
Cherries, maraschino	**12**	1 cherry	3	trace	low

Food	kCl/portion	Portion size	Carbs g	Fat g	Fibre
Cherry bakewells	206	1 individual cake	32	8	low
Cherry brandy	64	1 single measure	8	0	0
Cherry cheesecake	302	1 slice	41	13	low
Cherry compôte	78	3 heaped tbsp	20	trace	low
Cherry genoa cake	334	1 slice	51	12	medium
Cherry pie	282	1 slice	40	13	medium
Cherry pie filling	82	¼ large can	21	trace	low
Cherryade	18	1 tumbler	21	trace	0
Cheshire cheese	94	1 small wedge	trace	8	0
Chestnut purée, sweetened	45	1 tbsp	10	trace	medium
Chestnut purée, unsweetened	25	1 tbsp	5	trace	medium
Chestnut stuffing	58	1 serving	4	4	medium
Chestnuts	18	1 nut	4	trace	high
Chestnuts, peeled and cooked	65	5 nuts	14	trace	high
Chestnuts, roasted in shells	21	1 nut	4	trace	high
Chèvre cheese	80	1 small wedge	trace	7	0
Chewy cereal bars, all flavours	131 (avge)	1 bar	21	5	medium
Chick pea dahl	125	3 heaped tbsp	10	6	high
Chick pea goulash	338	1 serving	36	15	high
Chick peas (garbanzos), canned, drained	115	3 heaped tbsp	16	3	high

Food	kC/ portion	Carbs g	Fat g	Fibre
Chick peas, dried, soaked and boiled	121	18	2	high
Chicken, breast, cooked, sliced	35	0	1	0
Chicken, breast, grilled (broiled)	213	0	6	0
Chicken, breast, poached or steamed	244	0	7	0
Chicken, breast, smoked	23	trace	1	0
Chicken, breast portion, fried (sautéed), in breadcrumbs	363	22	19	low
Chicken, drumstick, barbecued	103	2	4	0
Chicken, drumstick, roast	92	0	3	0
Chicken, fried	494	19	29	low
Chicken, jerk	256	5	8	trace
Chicken, leg portion, barbecued	287	1	10	0
Chicken, leg portion, grilled	274	0	10	0
Chicken, leg portion, roast	276	0	10	0
Chicken, lemon	356	3	13	0
Chicken, minced (ground), stewed	183	0	7	0
Chicken, roast, with skin	216	0	14	0
Chicken, roast, without skin	148	0	5	0
Chicken, steamed	197	7	4	low

Portion size column:
- Chick peas, dried, soaked and boiled: 3 heaped tbsp
- Chicken, breast, cooked, sliced: 1 slice
- Chicken, breast, grilled (broiled): 1 medium breast
- Chicken, breast, poached or steamed: 1 medium breast
- Chicken, breast, smoked: 1 slice
- Chicken, breast portion, fried (sautéed), in breadcrumbs: ¼ small chicken
- Chicken, drumstick, barbecued: 1 drumstick
- Chicken, drumstick, roast: 1 drumstick
- Chicken, fried: 2 pieces
- Chicken, jerk: 1 serving
- Chicken, leg portion, barbecued: ¼ small chicken
- Chicken, leg portion, grilled: ¼ small chicken
- Chicken, leg portion, roast: ¼ small chicken
- Chicken, lemon: 1 medium breast
- Chicken, minced (ground), stewed: 1 serving
- Chicken, roast, with skin: 3 medium slices
- Chicken, roast, without skin: 3 medium slices
- Chicken, steamed: ¼ small chicken

Food	kC/ portion	Portion size	Carbs g	Fat g	Fibre
Chicken, sweet and sour	165	1 serving	32	2	high
Chicken, tandoori	375	¼ small chicken	4	19	trace
Chicken, thai, with noodles	506	1 serving	59	15	high
Chicken, wing portion, grilled (broiled)	220	¼ small chicken	0	9	0
Chicken, wing portion, roast	222	¼ small chicken	0	9	0
Chicken, wings, barbecued, Chinese-style	70	1 wing	3	2	0
Chicken à la king	**255**	1 serving	20	9	medium
Chicken and almond soup, canned	**180**	2 ladlefuls	9	14	low
Chicken and sweetcorn (corn) chowder, home-made	**183**	**2 ladlefuls**	**16**	**3**	**medium**
Chicken and sweetcorn soup, canned	**84**	2 ladlefuls	12	2	low
Chicken and sweetcorn soup, instant	119	1 mug	16	6	low
Chicken and ham paste	**56**	1 tbsp	trace	4	0
Chicken and ham pie, cold	**380**	1 slice	32	22	low
Chicken and mushroom casserole	**413**	1 serving	29	16	low
Chicken and mushroom chowder	**192**	2 ladlefuls	17	10	low

Food	kC/ portion	Portion size	Carbs g	Fat g	Fibre
Chicken and mushroom pie	246	1 individual pie	17	12	low
Chicken and mushroom soup, canned	76	2 ladlefuls	7	4	low
Chicken and mushroom soup, instant	58	1 mug	9	2	low
Chicken and rice soup, canned	82	2 ladlefuls	15	2	low
Chicken and rice soup, home–made	127	2 ladlefuls	13	3	low
Chicken and tarragon soup, home–made	116	2 ladlefuls	9	8	low
Chicken and vegetable soup, canned	82	2 ladlefuls	12	2	medium
Chicken and vegetable soup, home–made	165	2 ladlefuls	19	5	high
Chicken and vegetable stir–fry	270	1 serving	39	7	high
Chicken broth	64	2 ladlefuls	11	2	low
Chicken burger in a bun, home–made, with relish	366	1 burger in a bun	32	10	medium
Chicken burger sandwich	710	1 burger	54	43	medium
Chicken byriani	782	1 serving	75	38	medium
Chicken cacciatore	265	1 serving	36	4	high
Chicken casserole	374	1 serving	29	12	high

Food	kC/ portion	Portion size	Carbs g	Fat g	Fibre
Chicken chasseur	**440**	1 serving	67	7	medium
Chicken chop suey	**295**	1 serving	34	6	medium
Chicken chow mein	**337**	1 serving	28	5	high
Chicken cordon bleu	**344**	**1 serving**	**15**	**20**	**low**
Chicken curry, home-made	**615**	1 serving	9	51	medium
Chicken curry, home-made, with rice	**863**	1 serving	65	53	medium
Chicken curry, retail	**447**	1 serving	16	27	medium
Chicken curry, retail, with rice	**691**	1 serving	68	26	high
Chicken enchiladas	**566**	2 enchiladas	66	9	high
Chicken fajitas	**258**	2 fajitas	34	6	low
Chicken fingers	**27**	1 finger	2	1	low
Chicken fricassée	**280**	1 serving	6	16	medium
Chicken galantine	**268**	1 slice	9	14	medium
Chicken goujons	**162**	6 goujons	12	3	low
Chicken in black bean sauce	**221**	1 serving	10	6	medium
Chicken jalfrezi	**490**	1 serving	70	12	high
Chicken kiev	**473**	1 medium breast	22	31	low
Chicken korma	**460**	1 serving	16	21	medium
Chicken liver pâté	**158**	1 serving	trace	14	0
Chicken liver pâté, with toast and butter	**468**	1 serving plus 2 slices of toast	37	32	medium

Food	kC/ portion	Portion size	Carbs g	Fat g	Fibre
Chicken liver risotto	590	1 serving	89	27	low
Chicken livers, fried (sautéed)	194	1 serving	3	11	0
Chicken marsala	284	1 serving	2	5	low
Chicken maryland	484	¼ small chicken	30	25	low
Chicken mayonnaise sandwiches	458	1 round	34	41	medium
Chicken noodle soup, canned	50	2 ladlefuls	8	trace	low
Chicken noodle soup, home-made	145	2 ladlefuls	17	4	low
Chicken noodle soup, packet	40	2 ladlefuls	7	1	low
Chicken nuggets	253	6 nuggets	11	15	medium
Chicken omelette	293	2 eggs	trace	23	0
Chicken paprika	194	1 serving	6	7	low
Chicken paste	35	1 tbsp	trace	3	0
Chicken pie, individual	378	1 individual pie	30	22	low
Chicken pie, with puff pastry (paste)	572	1 serving	36	37	low
Chicken pot pie	485	1 slice	28	39	low
Chicken pot roast with vegetables	510	1 serving	65	11	high
Chicken ravioli	148	1 serving	26	1	medium
Chicken risotto	336	1 serving	83	8	low

Food	kCl/portion	Portion size	Carbs g	Fat g	Fibre
Chicken roll, sliced	22	1 slice	trace	1	0
Chicken salad	215	1 serving	5	7	high
Chicken salad, dressed	318	1 serving	5	19	high
Chicken sandwiches	341	1 round	34	23	medium
Chicken satay	172	1 stick	6	5	low
Chicken soup, cream of, canned	116	2 ladlefuls	9	8	0
Chicken soup, home-made	114	2 ladlefuls	7	4	0
Chicken soup, instant	100	1 mug	11	6	0
Chicken soup, low-fat, canned	44	2 ladlefuls	4	2	0
Chicken soup, packet	128	2 ladlefuls	21	5	0
Chicken stew with dumplings	537	1 serving	77	9	high
Chicken suprême	309	1 breast	8	12	low
Chicken tenders	350	8 pieces	17	22	low
Chicken teriyaki	317	1 serving	52	4	high
Chicken tikka	369	1 serving	11	17	medium
Chicken tikka masala	490	1 serving	44	18	high
Chicken véronique	254	1 serving	11	10	low
Chicken vindaloo	572	1 serving	7	40	medium
Chicory (Belgian endive)	18	1 head	trace	2	low
Chicory, braised	38	1 head	2	2	low

Food	kC/ portion	Portion size	Carbs g	Fat g	Fibre
Chilli beans	247	1 serving	52	2	high
Chilli con carne	302	1 serving	17	17	high
Chilli dog	204	1 dog in a bun	29	7	low
Chilli salsa	18	1 tbsp	4	trace	low
Chilli sauce	15	1 tbsp	3	trace	low
Chinese egg noodles, cooked	124	1 serving	26	1	medium
Chinese leaves (stem lettuce)	11	1 serving	1	0	low
Chinese pork spare ribs	310	2 ribs	13	17	low
Chipolata sausages, fried (sautéed)	61	1 sausage	2	5	low
Chipolata sausages, grilled (broiled)	58	1 sausage	2	5	low
Chips (fries), chip-shop	394	1 serving	49	20	high
Chips, crinkle-cut, frozen, deep-fried	478	1 serving	55	27	high
Chips, home-made, deep-fried	312	1 serving	50	11	high
Chips, microwave	221	1 small box	32	10	high
Chips, oven, frozen, baked	267	1 serving	49	7	high
Chips, straight-cut, frozen, deep-fried	450	1 serving	53	16	high
Chips, thin-cut	462	1 serving	56	26	high
See also French fries					

Food	kC/ portion	Portion size	Carbs g	Fat g	Fibre
Choc ice, any chocolate	180	1 ice cream	18	11	low
Choco corn flakes, dry	95	25 g/1 oz/½ cup	21	1	low
Choco corn flakes, with semi-skimmed milk	209	5 heaped tbsp	35	3	low
Choco corn flakes, with skimmed milk	193	5 heaped tbsp	35	1	low
Chocolate, milk	255	1 standard bar	28	14	0
Chocolate, plain (semi-sweet)	250	1 standard bar	30	13	0
Chocolate, white	109	1 standard (thin) bar	11	6	0
Chocolate, with fruit and nut	240	1 standard bar	27	12	0
Chocolate, with whole nuts	270	1 standard bar	24	17	0
Chocolate and walnut brownies	505	1 brownie	40	37	medium
Chocolate biscuits (cookies), full-coated	131	1 biscuit	17	7	low
Chocolate biscuits, half-coated	84	1 biscuit	11	4	low
Chocolate brazils	49	1 sweet (candy)	3	4	high
Chocolate brownies	368	1 brownie	63	11	medium
Chocolate buttons	175	1 small packet	19	10	0
Chocolate cake, chocolate-coated	268	1 slice	41	10	low
Chocolate cake, filled with butter cream	235	1 slice	35	10	low

Food	kC/ portion	Portion size	Carbs g	Fat g	Fibre
Chocolate caramels	25	1 sweet (candy)	6	trace	low
Chocolate cheesecake	271	1 slice	34	11	low
Chocolate chip chewy cereal bar	112	1 bar	17	4	low
Chocolate chip cookies	45	1 cookie	8	1	low
Chocolate chip ice cream	91	1 scoop	12	4	low
Chocolate chip muffin	397	1 muffin low			
Chocolate corn pops, dry	97	25 g/1 oz/½ cup	20	1	low
Chocolate corn pops, with semi-skimmed milk	213	5 heaped tbsp	38	4	low
Chocolate corn pops, with skimmed milk	197	5 heaped tbsp	38	2	low
Chocolate cream biscuits (cookies)	63	1 biscuit	9	3	low
Chocolate cream pie	343	1 slice	38	22	low
Chocolate crispix, dry	90	25 g/1 oz/½ cup	21	1	low
Chocolate crispix, with semi-skimmed milk	201	5 heaped tbsp	40	3	low
Chocolate crispix, with skimmed milk	185	5 heaped tbsp	40	1	low
Chocolate custard, canned	71	¼ large can	11	2	low
Chocolate dessert	136	1 individual pot	19	5	low
Chocolate dessert, with cream	225	1 individual pot	12	low	

Food	kC/ portion	Portion size	Carbs g	Fat g	Fibre
Chocolate digestives (graham crackers)	**88**	1 biscuit (cookie)	11	4	medium
Chocolate éclair toffees	**48**	1 toffee	7	2	low
Chocolate éclair, filled with cream	**277**	1 éclair	18	21	low
Chocolate éclair, filled with custard	**262**	1 éclair	24	16	low
Chocolate finger biscuits (cookies)	**38**	1 biscuit	5	2	low
Chocolate fudge	**65**	1 piece	13	1	low
Chocolate fudge cake	**420**	1 slice	70	14	low
Chocolate fudge fingers	**135**	1 finger	22	5	0
Chocolate fudge icing (frosting)	**77**	1 tbsp	9	1	low
Chocolate ginger	**30**	1 piece	7	trace	low
Chocolate ice cream	**89**	1 scoop	12	4	low
Chocolate layer cake	**384**	1 slice	58	14	low
Chocolate mini roll	**119**	1 roll	16	5	low
Chocolate mint creams	**39**	1 mint	8	1	0
Chocolate mousse	**139**	1 individual pot	10	5	0
Chocolate mousse, low-calorie	**88**	1 individual pot	0	3	0
Chocolate nut sundae	**417**	1 sundae	52	23	low

Food	kCl/portion	Portion size	Carbs g	Fat g	Fibre
Chocolate peanuts	200	1 small packet	19	13	medium
Chocolate pot	136	1 individual pot	19	5	low
Chocolate profiteroles	373	1 serving	33	24	medium
Chocolate pudding	340	1 serving	45	16	medium
Chocolate raisins	185	1 small packet	32	7	high
Chocolate ripple ice-cream	89	1 scoop	12	4	low
Chocolate roulade	206	1 serving	20	12	0
Chocolate sauce, for ice cream	192	2 tbsp	29	6	low
Chocolate sauce, made with semi-skimmed milk	112	5 tbsp	14	5	low
Chocolate sauce, made with skimmed milk	102	5 tbsp	14	4	low
Chocolate shreddies, dry	91	25 g/1 oz/½ cup	20	trace	medium
Chocolate shreddies, with semi-skimmed milk	224	5 heaped tbsp	42	3	high
Chocolate shreddies, with skimmed milk	208	5 heaped tbsp	42	1	high
Chocolate soufflé	103	1 serving	17	1	low
Chocolate soya ice dessert	52	1 scoop	5	3	0
Chocolate spread, all types	82 (avge)	1 tbsp1	9	5	low
Chocolate spread, with peanut butter	89	1 tbsp	5	7	medium

Food	kC/ portion	Portion size	Carbs g	Fat g	Fibre
Chocolate wafer bar	**115**	1 standard bar	13	6	0
Chocolates, assorted, filled	**46** (avge)	1 chocolate	7	2	0
Chorizo sausage	**273**	1 small sausage	1	23	0
Choux buns, filled with cream	**237**	1 bun	8	21	low
Choux buns, filled with custard	**293**	1 bun	27	17	low
Christmas cake, with marzipan and royal icing (frosting)	**356**	1 slice	63	11	medium
Christmas pudding	**291**	1 serving	49	10	medium
Ciabatta bread	**125**	1 medium slice	26	trace	medium
Cider, dry	**108**	1 small	8	0	0
Cider, medium–sweet	**126**	1 small	13	0	0
Cider, vintage	**303**	1 small	22	0	0
Cider cup	**62**	1 wine glass	17	0	0
Cigarettes russes	**56**	1 biscuit (cookie)	6	3	low
Cinnamon danish pastries	**270**	1 pastry	52	18	medium
Cinnamon grahams, dry	**102**	25 g/1 oz/½ cup	19	2	medium
Cinnamon grahams, with semi-skimmed milk	**182**	3 heaped tbsp	29	5	medium
Cinnamon grahams, with skimmed milk	**166**	3 heaped tbsp	29	3	medium
Clafoutis	**242**	1 serving	33	10	medium

Food	kC/ portion	Portion size	Carbs g	Fat g	Fibre
Clam bisque, canned	**85**	2 ladlefuls	12	2	low
Clam chowder, home-made	**253**	2 ladlefuls	17	10	medium
Clams, canned, drained	**60**	½ medium can	2	1	0
Clams, fresh, shelled, cooked	**93**	1 serving	4	1	0
Classic chocolate bar	**125**	1 standard bar	**15**	**7**	**low**
Clear conserve See *Jelly, individual flavours, e.g.* Mint jelly, Redcurrant jelly					
Clementine	**28**	1 fruit	6	trace	medium
Clotted cream fudge	**80**	1 square	14	3	0
Club chocolate bar, all flavours	**125** (avge)	1 bar	16	7	low
Clusters, dry	**97**	25 g/1 oz/½ cup	17	2	medium
Clusters, with skimmed milk	**160**	3 heaped tbsp	26	3	medium
Clusters, with semi-skimmed milk	**176**	3 heaped tbsp	26	5	medium
Cob loaf	**70**	1 medium slice	15	1	low
Cob nuts, shelled	**162**	25 g/1 oz/¼ cup	1	16	medium
Cobbler See individual *flavours, e.g.* Fruit cobbler					
Coca-cola	**78**	1 tumbler	21	0	0
Coca-cola, diet	**1**	1 tumbler	0	0	0

Food	kC/ portion	Portion size	Carbs g	Fat g	Fibre
Cock-a-leekie soup, home-made	**138**	2 ladlefuls	15	8	low
Cockles, fresh, shelled, cooked	48	1 serving	trace	trace	0
Cockles, preserved in vinegar	49	1 serving	1	trace	0
Cocktail sauce	51	1 tbsp	2	4	low
Coco pops, dry	95	25 g/1 oz/½ cup	21	1	low
Coco pops, with semi-skimmed milk	209	5 heaped tbsp	27	3	low
Coco pops, with skimmed milk	193	5 heaped tbsp	27	1	low
Coco pops cereal and milk bar	90	1 bar	14	3	low
Cocoa, made with semi-skimmed milk and sugar	142	1 mug	17	5	low
Cocoa, made with skimmed milk and sugar	126	1 mug	17	3	low
Coconut	330	¼ nut	13	31	high
Coconut, desiccated (shredded)	43	1 tbsp	1	9	high
Coconut cake	175	1 slice	20	19	low
Coconut ice sweet (candy) bar	464	1 standard bar	83	13	high
Coconut macaroons	117	1 macaroon	16	5	medium
Coconut pyramid	230	1 pyramid	42	6	high
Coconut rings/thins	35	1 biscuit (cookie)	5	1	low
Cod, baked	168	1 piece of fillet	0	2	0

Food	kCl/portion	Portion size	Carbs g	Fat g	Fibre
Cod, grilled (broiled)	166	1 piece of fillet	0	2	0
Cod, fried (sautéed), in batter	497	1 piece of fillet	19	26	low
Cod, fried (sautéed), in breadcrumbs	435	1 piece of fillet	9	21	low
Cod, salt, soaked and cooked	241	1 piece of fillet	0	2	0
Cod, with butter sauce	159	1 steak	9	9	low
Cod, with cheese sauce	175	1 steak	9	6	low
Cod, with mushroom sauce	168	1 steak	9	8	low
Cod, with parsley sauce	170	1 steak	11	5	low
Cod and prawn pie	328	1 individual pie	24	21	low
Cod mornay	415	1 steak	23	23	low
Cod provençal	273	1 serving	9	9	medium
Cod roes, in breadcrumbs, fried (sautéed)	202	1 serving	3	12	low
Cod roes, on toast	307	1 serving plus0 1 slice of toast	0	20	low
Coffee, black	5	1 mug	1	trace	0
Coffee, espresso	4	1 small cup	1	trace	0
Coffee, white, made with water and semi-skimmed milk	15	1 mug	2	trace	0
Coffee, white, made with water and skimmed milk	12	1 mug	2	trace	0

Food	kCl/portion	Portion size	Carbs g	Fat g	Fibre
Coffee and walnut cake	344	1 slice	34	19	medium
Coffee cake	258	1 slice	34	11	low
Coffee cheesecake	272	1 slice	30	13	low
Coffee granita	44	1 serving	11	trace	0
Coffee ice cream	89	1 scoop	12	4	low
Coffee mousse	139	1 serving	20	5	0
Coffee roulade	206	1 slice	20	12	0
Coffee streusel cake	263	1 slice	29	15	medium
Coffeemate	27	1 tsp	3	2	0
Coffeemate, light	21	1 tsp	3	1	0
Cointreau	78	1 single measure	7	0	0
Cola	78	1 tumbler	21	0	0
Cola, low-calorie	1	1 tumbler	0	0	0
Colcannon	240	1 serving	7	18	high
Coleslaw, home-made	92	2 tbsp	13	4	high
Coleslaw, low-calorie	28	2 tbsp	2	2	medium
Coleslaw, ready-made	40	2 tbsp	3	3	medium
Coley (sautéed), in batter	490	1 piece of fillet	19	25	low
Coley, fried, in breadcrumbs	428	1 piece of fillet	9	20	low
Coley, poached or steamed	147	1 piece of fillet	0	1	0

Food	kC/ portion	Portion size	Carbs g	Fat g	Fibre
Collard greens See Spring greens					
Complan, savoury, made with water	194	1 mug	24	7	0
Complan, sweet, made with semi-skimmed milk	260	1 mug	34	9	low
Complan, sweet, made with skimmed milk	240	1 mug	34	6	low
Complan, sweet, made with water	192	1 mug	27	6	low
Conchiglie (pasta shapes), dried, boiled	198	1 serving	42	1	medium
Conchiglie, fresh, boiled	235	1 serving	45	2	medium
Condensed milk, skimmed, sweetened	267	100 ml/3½ fl oz/ scant ½ cup	60	trace	0
Condensed milk, skimmed, unsweetened	80	100 ml/3½ fl oz/ scant ½ cup	11	trace	0
Condensed milk, whole, sweetened	333	100 ml/3½ fl oz/ scant ½ cup	55	10	0
Condensed milk, whole, unsweetened	151	100 ml/3½ fl oz/ scant ½ cup	8	9	0
Conger eel, grilled (broiled)	375	1 steak	0	24	0
Consommé, canned	14	2 ladlefuls	1	trace	0

Food	kC/ portion	Portion size	Carbs g	Fat g	Fibre
Consommé, jellied	32	2 ladlefuls	2	trace	0
Cookies See Biscuits					
Cook-in sauces, all flavours	**43** (avge)	1 serving	8	1	low
Coq au vin	**410**	1 serving	7	29	low
Coquilles st jacques	**212**	1 serving	20	10	medium
Cordial See individual flavours, e.g. Blackcurrant cordial					
Corn chips	**229**	1 small bag	30	11	medium
Corn chowder	**143**	2 ladlefuls	28	2	high
Corn cobs, baby, canned, drained	**23**	4 cobs	2	trace	medium
Corn cobs, baby, steamed or boiled	**24**	4 cobs	3	trace	medium
Corn cobs, baby, stir-fried	**69**	4 cobs	3	5	medium
Corn flakes, dry	**92**	25 g/1 oz/½ cup	20	trace	low
Corn flakes, with semi-skimmed milk	**149**	5 heaped tbsp	27	2	low
Corn flakes, with skimmed milk	**133**	5 heaped tbsp	27	trace	low
Corn flakes cereal and chocolate milk bar	**118**	1 bar	18	4	low
Corn fritters	**91**	1 fritter	16	2	medium

Food	kCl/portion	Portion size	Carbs g	Fat g	Fibre
Corn kernels, canned, drained See also *Sweetcorn*	122	3 heaped tbsp	27	1	medium
Corn pops, dry	90	25 g/1 oz/½ cup	22	trace	low
Corn pops, with semi-skimmed milk	209	5 heaped tbsp	38	3	low
Corn pops, with skimmed milk	193	5 heaped tbsp	38	1	low
Corn pops, chocolate, dry	97	25 g/1 oz/½ cup	20	1	low
Corn pops, chocolate, with semi-skimmed milk	213	5 heaped tbsp	38	4	low
Corn pops, chocolate, with skimmed milk	197	5 heaped tbsp	38	2	low
Corn puff snacks, all flavours	259 (avge)	1 small bag	27	16	low
Corn salad	3	1 handful	trace	trace	low
Cornbread	153	1 piece	22	5	medium
Corned beef	54	1 slice	0	3	0
Corned beef hash	387	1 serving	22	24	medium
Cornetto, all flavours	198 (avge)	1 cornet	26	10	medium
Cornflour pudding	134	1 serving	26	2	low
Cornichons See *Gherkins*					
Cornish crab soup, canned	118	2 ladlefuls	25	trace	low

Food	kC/ portion	Portion size	Carbs g	Fat g	Fibre
Cornish hen See Poussin					
Cornish ice cream	80	1 scoop	6	2	0
Cornish pasties	515	1 pasty	48	32	medium
Cornish wafers	47	1 wafer	5	3	low
Cornmeal See Polenta					
Cornmeal muffins	154	1 muffin	23	6	low
Cornmeal pancakes	97	1 pancake	15	3	low
Corn on the cob, steamed or boiled	99	1 cob	17	2	medium
Corn on the cob, with butter	173	1 cob	17	10	medium
Corn on the cob, with low-fat spread	138	1 cob	17	6	medium
Coronation chicken	266	1 serving	15	5	low
Cottage cheese	98	1 small tub	2	4	0
Cottage cheese, flavoured	95	1 small tub	3	4	0
Cottage cheese, low-fat	78	1 small tub	3	1	0
Cottage cheese, low-fat, flavoured	75	1 small tub	3	1	0
Cottage loaf	74	1 medium slice	15	1	low
Cottage pie	330	1 serving	25	19	medium
Coulibiac	380	1 thick slice	30	25	low
Country store, dry	87	25 g/1 oz/¼ cup	17	1	medium

Food	kC/portion	Portion size	Carbs g	Fat g	Fibre
Country store, with semi-skimmed milk	197	3 heaped tbsp	33	4	high
Country store, with skimmed milk	181	3 heaped tbsp	33	2	high
Courgettes (zucchini), fried (sautéed)	63	3 heaped tbsp	3	5	medium
Courgettes, steamed or boiled	19	3 heaped tbsp	2	trace	medium
Courgettes, stuffed	134	2 halves	12	8	medium
Courgettes provençal	69	3 heaped tbsp	8	3	medium
Couscous	177	3 heaped tbsp	29	4	medium
Couscous salad	159	3 heaped tbsp	23	6	high
Crab, dressed	459	1 medium crab	17	16	low
Crab, dressed, canned	21	½ small can	0	3	0
Crab, white meat	81	½ small can	0	1	0
Crab and mayonnaise sandwiches	447	1 round	34	29	medium
Crab bisque, home-made	185	2 ladlefuls	26	7	low
Crab cakes	93	1 cake	trace	4	0
Crab cocktail	102	1 serving	7	3	medium
Crab sandwiches	344	1 round	34	18	medium
Crabapple jelly (clear conserve)	55	1 tbsp	13	trace	0
Crabsticks	12	1 stick	1	trace	0

Food	kC/ portion	Portion size	Carbs g	Fat g	Fibre
Cracked wheat See Bulgar					
Crackerbread	20	1 piece	4	trace	low
Crackers, wholemeal See also Biscuits and individual names, e.g. Ritz	29	1 cracker	5	1	medium
Cranberries, dried	48	1 small handful	12	trace	high
Cranberries, stewed with sugar	70	3 heaped tbsp	18	trace	low
Cranberry jelly (clear conserve)	38	1 tbsp	10	0	low
Cranberry juice drink	104	1 tumbler	25	0	0
Cranberry juice drink, light	48	1 tumbler	11	0	0
Cranberry sauce	24	1 tbsp	6	0	low
Crayfish, boiled	148	½ crayfish	0	2	0
Cream, aerosol	46	1 tbsp	trace	5	0
Cream, canned	36	1 tbsp	trace	4	0
Cream, clotted	88	1 tbsp	trace	9	0
Cream, double (heavy)	67	1 tbsp	trace	7	0
Cream, half	22	1 tbsp	1	2	0
Cream, single (light)	30	1 tbsp	1	3	0
Cream, soured (dairy sour)	31	1 tbsp	1	3	0
Cream, sweetened, imitation	28	1 tbsp	1	4	0
Cream, whipping	56	1 tbsp	trace	6	0

Food	kC/ portion	Portion size	Carbs g	Fat g	Fibre
Cream cake	**337**	1 individual cake	43	17	low
Cream cheese	**110**	1 heaped tbsp	trace	12	0
Cream crackers	**39**	1 cracker	6	1	low
Cream crowdie	**691**	1 serving	14	52	medium
Cream of wheat See Semolina					
Cream soda	**58**	1 tumbler	14	trace	low
Cream soups, canned, all flavours	**110** (avge)	2 ladlefuls	9	8	low
See also individual entries, e.g. Cream of tomato soup					
Crème brûlée	**492**	1 serving	18	50	0
Crème caramel	**136**	1 individual po	26	2	0
Crème de cassis	**65**	1 single measure	7	0	0
Crème de menthe	**125**	1 single measure	14	trace	0
Crème egg, chocolate	**163**	1 egg	28	6	0
Crème fraîche	**56**	1 tbsp	trace	6	0
Crème fraîche, low-fat	**25**	1 tbsp	1	2	0
Crêpe, plain	**122**	1 crêpe	14	7	low
Crêpes suzette	**317**	2 pancakes	28	12	medium
Crispbread, rye	**27**	1 cracker	6	trace	medium
Crispbread, starch-reduced	**15**	1 cracker	3	trace	low
Crispbread, wheat	**35**	1 cracker	7	trace	low

Food	kC/ portion	Portion size	Carbs g	Fat g	Fibre
Crispie cakes	**69**	1 cake	11	3	low
Crisps (potato chips), all flavours	**136** (avge)	1 small bag	12	9	medium
Crisps, low-fat, all flavours	**114** (avge)	1 small bag	16	5	medium
Crispy chicken sandwich	**500**	1 portion	54	27	medium
Crispy chicken strips	**300**	3 strips	18	16	low
Crispy duck with pancakes	**665**	1 serving plus 6 pancakes	32	42	high
Crispy noodles	**374**	1 serving	50	17	low
Crispy vegetable fingers	**45**	1 finger	5	2	low
Croissant, all-butter	**185**	1 croissant	20	10	low
Croissant, apple	**144**	1 croissant	21	5	medium
Croissant, chocolate	**236**	1 croissant	26	13	low
Croissant, mini	**140**	1 croissant	15	8	low
Croissant, raisin	**212**	1 croissant	27	10	medium
Croque monsieur	**438**	1 round	36	27	medium
Croquette potatoes, fried (sautéed)	**214**	2 croquettes	22	13	medium
Croquette potatoes, frozen, baked	**90**	2 croquettes	14	3	low
Crostini, garlic	**31**	1 slice	5	1	low

Food	kC/ portion	Portion size	Carbs g	Fat g	Fibre
Crostini, mushroom	92	1 slice	16	2	low
Croûtons	75	1 tbsp	7	5	low
Crown roast of lamb	488	2 cutlets	0	40	0
Crudités	35	1 good handful	8	0	medium
Crudités, with aioli	272	1 serving	8	23	medium
Crumpet	80	1 crumpet	10	0	low
Crumpet, toasted, with butter	117	1 crumpet	10	4	low
Crumpet, toasted, with low-fat spread	99	1 crumpet	10	2	low
Crunchie chocolate bar	195	1 standard bar	30	8	0
Crunchy bran, dry	74	25 g/1 oz/½ cup	13	1	high
Crunchy bran, with semi-skimmed milk	175	5 heaped tbsp	27	4	high
Crunchy bran, with skimmed milk	159	5 heaped tbsp	27	2	high
Crunchy cereal bars, all flavours	146 (avge)	1 bar	17	7	medium
Crunchy mixed grain cereal, with nuts and raisins, dry	97	25 g/1 oz/¼ cup	16	3	high
Crunchy mixed grain cereal, with nuts and raisins and semi-skimmed milk	250	3 heaped tbsp9	37	7	high

Food	kCl/portion	Portion size	Carbs g	Fat g	Fibre
Crunchy mixed grain cereal, with nuts and raisins and skimmed milk	234	3 heaped tbsp	37	5	high
Crunchy nut corn flakes, dry	97	25 g/1 oz/½ cup	20	1	low
Crunchy nut corn flakes, with semi-skimmed milk	213	5 heaped tbsp	39	3	low
Crunchy nut corn flakes, with skimmed milk	197	5 heaped tbsp	39	1	low
Cucumber	4	5 slices	1	0	low
Cucumber and yoghurt soup	78	2 ladlefuls	9	3	low
Cucumber sandwiches	308	1 round	35	17	medium
Cullen skink	170	2 ladlefuls	16	6	low
Cumberland butter	53	1 tbsp	29	22	0
Cumberland sauce	64	1 tbsp	14	trace	0
Cumberland sausage, fried (sautéed)	317	1 sausage	11	24	low
Cupcakes, iced (frosted)	179	1 cake	37	3	low
Curaçao	78	1 single measure	7	0	0
Curd cheese	30	1 heaped tbsp	trace	12	0
Curd, lemon or orange	42	1 tbsp	9	1	low
Curly endive (frisée)	6	1 good handful	2	trace	medium
Curly kale, steamed or boiled	24	3 heaped tbsp	1	1	medium

Food	kC/ portion	Portion size	Carbs g	Fat g	Fibre
Curly wurly chocolate bar	**125**	1 standard bar	20	5	0
Currant bread	**72**	1 slice	13	2	low
Currant bread, with butter	146	1 slice	13	10	low
Currant bread, with low-fat spread	**111**	1 slice	13	6	low
Currant bun	**148**	1 bun	26	4	medium
Currant bun, with butter	**222**	1 bun	26	12	medium
Currant bun, with low-fat spread	**187**	1 bun	26	8	medium
Currant cake	**177**	1 slice	29	6	medium
Currants	**40**	1 small handful	10	trace	high
Curried beans	**168**	1 small can	31	1	high
Curried chicken and rice salad	**390**	1 serving	43	6	high
Curried fruit chutney	**19**	1 tbsp	4	trace	low
Curry sauce	**58**	5 tbsp	5	4	low
Custard, canned/carton	**71**	5 tbsp	11	2	low
Custard, chocolate	**71**	5 tbsp	11	2	low
Custard, egg, baked	**130**	1 serving	12	7	0
Custard, made with powder and semi-skimmed milk	**75**	5 tbsp	13	trace	low
Custard, made with powder and skimmed milk	**59**	5 tbsp	13	2	low

Food	kC/ portion	Portion size	Carbs g	Fat g	Fibre
Custard apple	**101**	1 fruit	25	1	medium
Custard creams	**57**	1 biscuit (cookie)	8	3	low
Custard sauce, made with semi-skimmed milk	**62**	5 tbsp	7	2	0
Custard sauce, made with skimmed milk	**52**	5 tbsp	7	1	0
Custard tart	**373**	1 individual tart	44	20	medium
Custard-style yoghurt	**161**	1 individual pot	3	13	0
Cuttlefish, grilled (broiled)	**278**	1 serving	2	2	0

Food	kC/ portion	Portion size	Carbs g	Fat g	Fibre
Dab, fried (sautéed) in breadcrumbs	378	1 medium fish	16	23	low
Dab, grilled (broiled)	175	1 medium fish	0	3	0
Daiquiri	111	1 cocktail	4	0	0
Dairy milk chocolate bar	255	1 standard bar	28	14	0
Daktyla bread	65	1 medium slice	12	1	medium
Damsons	3	1 fruit	1	trace	medium
Damsons, stewed	27	3 heaped tbsp	6	trace	medium
Damsons, stewed with sugar	107	3 heaped tbsp	19	trace	medium
Damson jam (conserve)	39	1 tbsp	10	0	0
Damson pie	290	1 slice	14	39	medium
Dandelion and burdock	56	1 tumbler	13	trace	low
Dandelion and burdock, low-calorie	3	1 tumbler	0	0	0
Danish apple cake	252	1 slice	32	10	high
Danish blue cheese	87	1 small wedge	trace	7	0
Danish brown bread	51	1 medium slice	10	trace	medium
Danish elbo cheese	86	1 small wedge	trace	7	0
Danish lumpfish roe	40	1 tbsp	1	3	0
Danish pastries, all types	374 (avge)	1 pastry	51	18	medium
Danish toaster bread	65	1 slice	12	1	low

Food	kC/ portion	Portion size	Carbs g	Fat g	Fibre
Danish toaster bread, toasted, with butter	129	1 slice	12	9	low
Danish toaster bread, toasted, with low-fat spread	94	1 slice	12	5	low
Danish white bread	50	1 medium slice	10	trace	low
Date squares	170	1 square	32	4	high
Dates	30	1 fruit	8	trace	high
Dates, dried	40	1 fruit	10	trace	high
Dates, stuffed	50	1 fruit	12	4	high
Dauphinoise potatoes	235	1 serving	12	15	medium
Derby cheese	100	1 small wedge	trace	8	0
Devilled chicken	309	1 serving	6	12	0
Devilled kidneys	158	1 serving	2	7	0
Devil's food cake	255	1 slice	40	8	low
Devils on horseback	52	1 roll	3	4	low
Dhal	162	3 heaped tbsp	21	6	high
Diet coke	1	1 tumbler	0	0	0
Diet pepsi	1	1 tumbler	trace	trace	0
Digestive biscuits (graham crackers)	73	1 biscuit (cookie)	10	3	low
Digestive caramels, chocolate	81	1 biscuit	11	4	medium
Digestive creams	63	1 biscuit (cookie)	8	3	low

Food	kC/ portion	Portion size	Carbs g	Fat g	Fibre
Dijon mustard	8	1 tsp	trace	trace	low
Dill pickled cucumbers	15	1 pickle	3	trace	low
Dim sum, assorted	49 (avge)	1 piece	6	2	low
Ditali (pasta shapes), dried, boiled	198	1 serving	42	1	medium
Ditali, fresh, boiled	235	1 serving	45	2	medium
Dogfish, fried (sautéed), in batter	464	1 piece of fillet	13	33	low
Dolcelatte cheese	106	1 small wedge	trace	10	0
Dolmas	221	2 rolls	19	9	high
Donor kebab, in pitta bread	588	1 kebab plus 1 bread	32	38	medium
Dorset blue cheese	87	1 small wedge	trace	7	0
Double chocolate chip muffin	397	1 muffin	48	20	low
Double decker chocolate bar	235	1 bar	32	10	0
Double gloucester cheese	101	1 small wedge	trace	8	0
Doughnut, apple	243	1 doughnut	29	12	low
Doughnut, chocolate	270	1 doughnut	26	18	medium
Doughnut, cream	265	1 doughnut	43	15	low
Doughnut, iced (frosted)	286	1 doughnut	42	12	low
Doughnut, jam (jelly)	252	1 doughnut	37	11	low
Doughnut, mini	59	1 doughnut	7	3	low

Food	kC/ portion	Portion size	Carbs g	Fat g	Fibre
Doughnut, plain, ring	236	1 doughnut	27	12	low
Dover sole, fried (sautéed), in seasoned flour	342	1 medium fish	8	13	low
Dover sole, grilled (broiled)	202	1 medium fish	0	9	0
Dr pepper soft drink	78	1 tumbler	21	0	0
Dr pepper, diet	1	1 tumbler	0	0	0
Drambuie	85	1 single measure	7	0	0
Dream topping, made with semi-skimmed milk	75	3 heaped tbsp	5	6	low
Dream topping, made with skimmed milk	66	3 heaped tbsp	5	4	low
Dream topping, sugar-free, made with semi-skimmed milk	75	3 heaped tbsp	5	5	low
Dream topping, sugar-free, made with skimmed milk	70	3 heaped tbsp	5	3	low
Dressed crab	459	1 medium crab	17	16	low
Dressed crab, canned	21	½ small can	0	3	0
Dried fruit compôte	127	3 heaped tbsp	33	trace	high
Drifter chocolate bar	292	1 standard bar	40	13	low
Drinking (sweetened) chocolate, made with semi-skimmed milk	177	1 mug	27	5	low

Food	kCl portion	Portion size	Carbs g	Fat g	Fibre
Drinking chocolate, made with skimmed milk	**146**	1 mug	27	1	low
Drinking chocolate, instant, made with water	**119**	1 mug	18	4	low
Drinking yoghurt	**124**	1 tumbler	26	trace	0
Drop scone (small pancake)	**44**	1 pancake	6	2	low
Dry-cured Belgian ham	**21**	1 slice	0	1	0
Dry-roasted peanuts	**88**	1 small handful	1	7	high
Dublin bay prawns (saltwater crayfish), cooked	**10**	1 prawn	0	trace	0
Dubonnet, red	**75**	1 double measure	8	0	0
Duchesse potatoes	**165**	2 pieces	17	5	medium
Duck, breast, grilled (broiled), without skin	**378**	1 breast	0	19	0
Duck, breast, grilled, with skin	**678**	1 breast	0	58	0
Duck, crispy peking	**665**	1 serving plus 6 pancakes	32	42	high
Duck, roast, with skin	**763**	¼ duck	0	65	0
Duck à l'orange	**856**	¼ duck	8	69	medium
Duck eggs, boiled	**106**	1 egg	trace	8	0
Duck liver pâté	**158**	1 serving	trace	14	0
Duck soup, home-made	**114**	2 ladlefuls	4	0	

Food	kC/ portion	Portion size	Carbs g	Fat g	Fibre
Duck with cherries	**836**	¼ duck	4	65	low
Dumplings	**73**	1 dumpling	9	1	low
Dundee cake	**397**	1 slice	58	17	medium
Dunlop cheese	**103**	1 small wedge	trace	9	0
Dutch apple tart	**237**	1 slice	34	10	medium

Food	kC/ portion	Portion size	Carbs g	Fat g	Fibre
Easter biscuits (cookies)	58	1 biscuit	16	4	low
Eccles cake	214	1 cake	26	12	medium
Echo chocolate bar	132	1 standard bar	15	7	low
Eclair, chocolate	277	1 éclair	18	21	low
Edam (dutch) cheese	83	1 small wedg	trace	6	0
Eel pie mash, with pea gravy	434	1 serving	35	25	medium
Eels, jellied	70	1 small serving	trace	6	0
Eels, silver, stewed	320	1 serving	0	13	0
Eels, smoked	167	1 serving	0	13	0
Egg, baked, with cream	151	1 egg	trace	13	0
Egg, boiled	84	1 egg	trace	6	0
Egg, coddled	84	1 egg	trace	6	0
Egg, curried	226	2 eggs	5	16	low
Egg, fried (sautéed)	102	1 egg	trace	8	0
Egg, pickled	84	1 egg	trace	6	0
Egg, poached	84	1 egg	trace	6	0
Egg, scotch	301	1 egg	16	20	low
Egg, scrambled	308	2 eggs	1	28	0
Egg, stuffed	187	2 halves	trace	17	0
Egg and cress sandwiches	392	1 round	68	23	medium
Egg custard tart	373	1 individual tart	44	20	medium

Food	kCl/portion	Portion size	Carbs g	Fat g	Fibre
Egg custard, baked	**130**	1 serving	12	7	0
Egg custard, packet, made up with semi-skimmed milk	**168**	1 serving	23	6	0
Egg custard, packet, made up with skimmed milk	**149**	1 serving	23	4	0
Egg fried rice	**374**	1 serving	46	19	low
Egg mayonnaise	**290**	1 egg	trace	29	0
Egg mayonnaise sandwiches	**491**	1 round	34	34	medium
Egg mcmuffin	**290**	1 portion	27	12	medium
Egg nog	**68**	1 single measure	7	2	0
Egg noodles, chinese	**124**	1 serving	26	1	medium
Egg salad	**200**	2 eggs	5	12	high
Egg salad, dressed	**297**	2 eggs	5	29	high
Egg sauce	**117**	5 tbsp	8	7	low
Eggplant *See Aubergine*					
Eggs benedict	**402**	1 egg	43	17	medium
Eggs florentine	**239**	1 egg	7	16	medium
Eggy bread	**213**	1 slice	17	18	low
Elderflower pressé	**50**	1 wine glass	12	trace	0
Elmlea cream blend, double (heavy)	**61**	1 tbsp	trace	6	low
Elmlea, single (light)	**48**	1 tbsp	trace	5	low

Food	kC/ portion	Portion size	Carbs g	Fat g	Fibre
Elmlea, whipping	43	1 tbsp	trace	4	low
Elmlea light, double (heavy)	37	1 tbsp	1	4	low
Elmlea light, single (light)	17	1 tbsp	trace	3	low
Elmlea light, whipping	28	1 tbspe	trace	2	low
Emmental (swiss) cheese	105	1 small wedge	1	8	0
Enchiladas *See individual fillings, e.g. Cheese enchiladas*					
English muffin	127	1 muffin	27	1	medium
English muffin, toasted, with butter	200	1 muffin	27	9	medium
English muffin, toasted, with low-fat spread	166	1 muffin	27	5	medium
English mustard	7	1 tsp	trace	trace	low
Escargots à la bourguignonne	311	6 snails	trace	25	low
Escarole	6	1 good handful	2	trace	medium
Esrom cheese	84	1 small wedge	trace	7	0
Evaporated milk	151	100 ml/3½ fl oz/ scant ½ cup	8	9	0
Evaporated milk, light	80	100 ml/3½ fl oz/ scant ½ cup	11	trace	0
Everton mints	21	1 mint	4	trace	0

Food	kC/portion	Portion size	Carbs g	Fat g	Fibre
Everton toffee	**20**	1 toffee	1	0	0
Eve's pudding	**222**	1 serving	40	6	medium
Exotic fruit drink	**90**	1 tumbler	22	trace	0

Food	kCl portion	Portion size	Carbs g	Fat g	Fibre
Fab ice lolly	**99**	1 lolly	17	3	0
Faggots	**402**	2 faggots	23	27	low
Fairy cakes	**105**	1 individual cake	22	2	low
Fajitas See *individual fillings, e.g. Beef fajitas*					
Falafels	**140**	2 falafels	11	9	high
Fanta orange	**85**	1 tumbler	22	0	0
Fanta orange, diet	**6**	1 tumbler	0	0	0
Farfalle (pasta shapes), dried, boiled	**198**	1 serving	42	1	medium
Farfalle, fresh, boiled	**235**	1 serving	45	2	medium
Farmhouse loaf	**74**	**1 medium slice**	**15**	**1**	**low**
Farmhouse vegetable soup, canned	**90**	2 ladlefuls	16	1	medium
Farmhouse vegetable soup, packet	**119**	2 ladlefuls	25	1	high
Feast ice lolly	**313**	1 lolly	23	13	low
Fennel	**27**	1 head	4	3	medium
Fennel, au gratin	**145**	1 serving	8	10	medium
Fennel, steamed or boiled	**11**	½ head	1	trace	medium
Feta cheese	**62**	1 small chunk	trace	5	0
Feta cheese, with olives	**19**	1 piece of each	trace	2	low

Food	kC/ portion	Portion size	Carbs g	Fat g	Fibre
Fettuccine (pasta ribbons), dried, boiled	**239**	1 serving	51	2	medium
Fettuccine, fresh, boiled	**301**	1 serving	57	2	medium
Fibre 1, dry	**66**	25 g/1 oz/½ cup	13	1	high
Fibre 1, with semi-skimmed milk	**166**	5 heaped tbsp	26	3	high
Fibre 1, with skimmed milk	**150**	5 heaped tbsp	26	1	high
Fig roll biscuit (cookie)	**61**	1 roll	11	2	medium
Figgy duff	**581**	1 serving	80	28	high
Figs	**24**	1 fig	5	trace	high
Figs, canned in syrup	**88**	3 heaped tbsp	25	trace	high
Figs, dried, ready-to-eat	**45**	1 fig	11	trace	high
Figs, dried, stewed	**103**	3 heaped tbsp	29	1	high
Figs, dried, stewed with sugar	**143**	3 heaped tbsp	34	1	high
Figs, with parma ham	**87**	1 fig plus 2 slices of ham	11	2	high
Filberts See Hazelnuts					
Filet-o-fish	**389**	1 portion	41	18	medium
Fillet steak See Steak, fillet					
Fingers, milk chocolate	**38**	1 biscuit (cookie)	6	1	low
Finger rolls	**107**	1 roll	21	2	low
Finnan haddie	**148**	1 fish	0	1	0

Food	kC/portion	Portion size	Carbs g	Fat g	Fibre
Fish and chips, deep-fried, chip-shop-style	891	1 serving	68	46	high
Fish cakes, salmon, fried (sautéed)	213	1 cake	15	11	low
Fish cakes, salmon, grilled (broiled)	192	1 cake	17	7	low
Fish cakes, white fish, fried	188	1 cake	15	10	low
Fish cakes, white fish, grilled	169	1 cake	17	6	low
Fish chowder	285	2 ladlefuls	60	10	medium
Fish fingers, fried (sautéed)	47	1 finger	3	3	low
Fish fingers, grilled (broiled)	43	1 finger	4	2	low
Fish goujons	304	6 goujons	6	14	low
Fish kebabs	95	1 kebab	0	1	0
Fish mornay	239	1 serving	13	21	low
Fish mousse	180	1 serving	6	15	low
Fish paste	25	1 tbsp	trace	1	low
Fish pie, topped with pastry (paste)	384	1 serving	27	25	low
Fish pie, topped with potato	315	1 serving	37	9	medium
Fish soup	159	2 ladlefuls	21	2	medium
Fish stew	330	1 serving	43	5	medium
Fish sticks	76	1 stick	7	3	0

Food	kC/ portion	Portion size	Carbs g	Fat g	Fibre
Flageolet beans, canned, drained	98	3 heaped tbsp	21	1	high
Flageolet beans, dried, soaked and cooked	104	3 heaped tbsp	23	1	high
Flake chocolate bar	180	1 standard bar	19	10	0
Flan, fruit, any flavour	222	1 slice	40	6	low
Flapjack	417	1 piece	48	23	high
Florida cocktail	56	1 serving	10	trace	low
Flounder, fried (sautéed)	378	1 small fish	16	23	low
Flounder, grilled (broiled)	175	1 small fish	0	2	0
Focaccia bread	139	1 medium slice	30	1	medium
Fois gras	158	1 serving	trace	14	0
Fondant creams	25	1 sweet (candy)	7	0	0
Fondant icing (frosting)	100	25 g/1 oz	25	0	0
Fondue, cheese	492	1 serving	8	29	0
Fondue, cheese, with French bread	762	1 serving plus 10 cubes of bread	62	31	medium
Fontina cheese	110	1 small wedge	trace	9	0
Forcemeat balls	115	2 balls	10	7	low
Four cheese pizza	334	1 slice	36	17	medium
Four cheese pasta sauce	500	¼ jar	76	13	medium
Four seasons pizza	342	1 slice	32	16	medium

Food	kC/ portion	Portion size	Carbs g	Fat g	Fibre
Framboise liqueur	**65**	1 single measure	7	0	0
Frankfurter	**186**	1 frankfurter	2	15	low
Frankfurter, canned	**82**	1 frankfurter	1	7	low
French (green) beans, canned, drained	**22**	3 heaped tbsp	4	trace	medium
French beans, steamed or boiled	**25**	3 heaped tbsp	5	trace	high
French dressing	**97**	1 tbsp	0	17	0
French dressing, low-calorie	**5**	1 tbsp	1	trace	0
French fancies, fondant-iced (frosted)	**150**	1 cake	25	5	low
French fries, thin, from burger outlets See also Chips	**206**	1 serving	28	9	medium
French mustard	**7**	1 tsp	1	trace	low
French onion soup, canned	**48**	2 ladlefuls	11	trace	low
French onion soup, home-made	**94**	2 ladlefuls	8	6	low
French onion soup, packet	**104**	2 ladlefuls	20	1	low
French onion soup, with cheese croûtes	**226**	2 ladlefuls plus 1 croûte	21	8	low
French stick	**135**	1 thick slice	27	1	low
French toast	**213**	1 slice	17	18	low

Food	kC/ portion	Portion size	Carbs g	Fat g	Fibre
Fried (sautéed) bread	181	1 slice	17	11	low
Fried (sautéed) egg sandwiches	406	1 round	34	25	medium
Fried rice See Rice, Egg fried rice *and* Special fried rice					
Fries See Chips					
Frisée See Curly endive					
Frito misto	338	1 serving	43	11	low
Frittata	328	2 eggs	17	22	medium
Frogs' legs, fried (sautéed)	178	2 legs	0	10	low
Fromage blanc	24	1 heaped tbsp	trace	trace	0
Fromage frais	113	1 individual pot	6	7	0
Fromage frais, flavoured	131	1 individual pot	14	6	low
Fromage frais, low-fat	58	1 individual pot	7	trace	low
Fromage frais, low-fat, flavoured	58	1 individual pot	7	trace	low
Frosted shreddies, dry	91	25 g/1 oz/½ cup	20	trace	high
Frosted shreddies, with semi-skimmed milk	224	5 heaped tbsp	43	3	high
Frosted shreddies, with skimmed milk	208	5 heaped tbsp	43	1	high
Frosted wheats, dry	80	25 g/1 oz/½ cup	17	trace	high

Food	kCl/ portion	Portion size	Carbs g	Fat g	Fibre
Frosted wheats, with semi-skimmed milk	**185**	5 heaped tbsp	34	3	high
Frosted wheats, with skimmed milk	**169**	5 heaped tbsp	34	1	high
Frosties, dry	**95**	25 g/1 oz/½ cup	22	trace	low
Frosties, with semi-skimmed milk	**209**	5 heaped tbsp	41	2	low
Frosties, with skimmed milk	**193**	5 heaped tbsp	41	trace	low
Frosties cereal and milk bar	**121**	1 bar	18	4	low
Frosting See **Icing**					
Fruit cake, light	**354**	1 slice	58	13	medium
Fruit cake, rich See *also* Christmas cake	**341**	1 slice	60	11	medium
Fruit chewy sweets (candies)	**185**	1 tube	38	4	0
Fruit cobbler	**255**	1 serving	46	7	medium
Fruit cocktail, canned in natural juice	**57**	3 heaped tbsp	15	trace	low
Fruit cocktail, canned in syrup	**77**	3 heaped tbsp	20	trace	low
Fruit corner yoghurt dessert	**219**	1 individual carton	26	7	low
Fruit flan, made with pastry (paste)	**153**	1 slice	24	6	low
Fruit flan, made with sponge	**222**	1 slice	40	1	low

Food	kC/ portion	Portion size	Carbs g	Fat g	Fibre
Fruit gums	**134**	1 tube	32	0	0
Fruit 'n' fibre, dry	**87**	25 g/1 oz/½ cup	17	1	high
Fruit 'n' fibre, with semi-skimmed milk	197	5 heaped tbsp	34	4	high
Fruit 'n' fibre, with skimmed milk	181	5 heaped tbsp	34	2	high
Fruit pastilles	**147**	1 tube	35	0	0
Fruit pie	**241**	1 individual pie	39	8	medium
Fruit punch	**59**	1 wine glass	15	0	low
Fruit salad, canned in natural juice	**29**	3 heaped tbsp	7	trace	low
Fruit salad, canned in syrup	57	3 heaped tbsp	15	trace	low
Fruit salad, dried	145	3 heaped tbsp	40	trace	high
Fruit salad, dried, stewed	83	3 heaped tbsp	26	trace	high
Fruit salad, dried, stewed with sugar	94	3 heaped tbsp	29	trace	high
Fruit salad, fresh, in pure juice	27	3 heaped tbsp	7	trace	medium
Fruit salad, fresh, in syrup	55	3 heaped tbsp	14	trace	medium
Fruit salad, tropical	47	3 heaped tbsp	9	0	medium
Fruit scone (biscuit)	**158**	1 scone	26	5	medium
Fruit scone, with butter	232	1 scone	26	13	medium

Food	kCl/portion	Portion size	Carbs g	Fat g	Fibre
Fruit scone, with low-fat spread	197	1 scone	26	9	medium
Fruit shortcake	52	1 biscuit (cookie)	7	2	low
Fruit squash See individual flavours, e.g. Orange squash					
Fruitful shredded wheat, dry	88	25 g/1 oz/½ cup	17	1	high
Fruitful shredded wheat, with semi-skimmed milk	202	3 heaped tbsp	34	4	high
Fruitful shredded wheat, with skimmed milk	186	3 heaped tbsp	34	2	high
Fruitibix, dry	88	25 g/1 oz/½ cup	18	1	high
Fruitibix, with semi-skimmed milk	200	3 heaped tbsp	34	3	high
Fruitibix, with skimmed milk	184	3 heaped tbsp	34	1	high
Fudge See also individual flavours, e.g. Chocolate fudge	77	1 square	14	2	0
Fudge brownie	394	1 brownie	62	20	low
Ful medames beans, dried, soaked and cooked	116	3 heaped tbsp	20	1	high
Fusilli (pasta spirals), dried, boiled	239	1 serving	51	2	medium
Fusilli, fresh, boiled	301	1 serving	57	2	medium

F

Food	kC/ portion	Portion size	Carbs g	Fat g	Fibre

Food	kC/ portion	Portion size	Carbs g	Fat g	Fibre
Gaelic coffee	218	1 wine glass	7	14	0
Gala pie	564	1 slice	37	68	medium
Galaxy chocolate bar, all flavours	250 (avge)	1 standard bar	27	14	0
Galaxy cake bar	178	1 cake bar	20	10	low
Galaxy cake bar, caramel	148	1 cake bar	20	7	low
Galaxy double nut and raisin bar	246	1 standard bar	26	14	0
Galaxy ice cream	302	1 ice cream bar	28	19	0
Galaxy muffin	356	1 muffin	42	18	low
Game chips	273	10 chips	25	19	medium
Game pie	606	1 serving	49	35	medium
Game soup, canned	88	2 ladlefuls	10	4	low
Gammon, honey-roast	174	2 thick slices	4	6	0
Gammon, lean, boiled	167	2 thick slices	0	5	0
Gammon, rasher (slice), fried (sautéed)	171	1 rasher	0	9	0
Gammon, rasher, grilled (broiled)	141	1 rasher	0	8	0
Gammon, steak, grilled	301	1 medium steak	0	9	0
Gammon with pineapple	324	1 medium steak plus 1 pineapple slice	6	9	medium

Food	kC/ portion	Portion size	Carbs g	Fat g	Fibre
Gammon and egg	**403**	1 medium steak plus 1 egg	trace	17	0
Garbanzos See Chick peas					
Garibaldi biscuits (cookies)	**41**	1 biscuit	7	1	low
Garlic	**5**	1 clove	1	trace	low
Garlic and herb soft cheese	**77**	1 good spoonful	1	7	low
Garlic bread	**73**	1 small slice	7	4	low
Garlic butter	**112**	1 tbsp	trace	12	low
Garlic chicken	**316**	1 breast	3	16	low
Garlic mayonnaise	**237**	2 tbsp	trace	23	0
Garlic sausage	**12**	1 slice	trace	1	low
Gazpacho	**136**	2 ladlefuls	trace	7	medium
Genoa cake	**383**	1 slice	56	16	medium
German smoked cheese	**60**	1 small wedge	trace	3	0
Ghee	**224**	25 g/1 oz/2 tbsp	trace	25	0
Gherkins (cornichons)	**4**	1 gherkin	1	trace	low
Gin	**55**	1 single measure	trace	0	0
Gin and dry martini	**114**	1 cocktail	3	trace	0
Gin and lime	**111**	1 single measure	15	0	0
Gin and orange	**108**	1 single measure	7	0	0
Gin and sweet martini	**130**	1 cocktail	8	0	0

Food	kC/ portion	Portion size	Carbs g	Fat g	Fibre
Gin and tonic	76	1 single measure plus 1 mixer	5	0	0
Gin and tonic, low-calorie	56	1 single measure plus 1 mixer	trace	trace	0
Ginger, chocolate	30	1 piece	7	trace	low
Ginger, crystallised	30	1 piece	4	0	low
Ginger, stem, in syrup	30	1 piece	2	trace	low
Ginger ale, american	44	1 tumbler	10	0	0
Ginger ale, dry	32	1 tumbler	8	0	0
Ginger ale, low-calorie	1	1 tumbler	trace	trace	0
Ginger beer	98	1 tumbler	24	0	0
Ginger cake	388	1 slice	60	15	medium
Ginger cake bar	128	1 cake bar	22	4	low
Ginger ice cream	89	1 scoop	11	4	low
Ginger nuts	56	1 biscuit (cookie)	9	2	low
Ginger nuts, milk or plain (semi-sweet) chocolate	70	1 biscuit	10	3	low
Ginger snaps	37	1 biscuit (cookie)	6	1	low
Ginger wine	200	1 double measure	16	0	0
Gingerbread	180	1 slice	28	7	low
Gingerbread men	249	1 man	34	11	low
Gipsy creams	64	1 biscuit (cookie)	8	3	low

Food	kC/ portion	Portion size	Carbs g	Fat g	Fibre
Gjetost cheese	**132**	1 small wedge	12	8	0
Glacé (candied) cherries	**13**	1 cherry	4	trace	low
Glacé (candied) fruits	**13**	1 piece	4	trace	low
Glacé icing (frosting)	**56**	1 tbsp	14	0	0
Globe artichoke, whole, steamed or boiled See also Artichokes	**70**	1 medium artichoke	3	0	medium
Globe artichoke heart, canned, drained	**8**	1 heart	1	trace	medium
Glucose, powdered or liquid	**48**	1 tbsp	13	0	0
Gnocchi	**213**	1 serving	13	12	low
Gnocchi, with butter and Parmesan	**385**	1 serving	13	29	low
Goats' cheese, hard	**128**	1 small wedge	1	10	0
Goats' cheese, soft	**152**	1 heaped tbsp	trace	12	0
Goats' milk	**180**	300 ml/½ pt/1¼ cups	12	10	0
Golden cutlets (smoked, whiting), poached	**166**	1 medium fillet	0	1	0
Golden grahams, dry	**93**	25 g/1 oz/½ cup	20	1	low
Golden grahams, with semi-skimmed milk	**172**	5 heaped tbsp	30	3	low
Golden grahams, with skimmed milk	**156**	5 heaped tbsp	30	1	low

Food	kC/ portion	Portion size	Carbs g	Fat g	Fibre
Golden nuggets, dry	95	25 g/1 oz/½ cup	22	trace	low
Golden nuggets, with semi-skimmed milk	174	5 heaped tbsp	32	2	low
Golden nuggets, with skimmed milk	158	5 heaped tbsp	32	trace	low
Golden raisins See Sultanas					
Golden (light corn) syrup	45	1 tbsp	12	0	0
Golden syrup cake bar	385	1 cake bar	60	14	medium
Golden syrup cake bar, mini	126	1 cake bar	22	4	low
Goose, roast, without skin	319	3 medium slices	0	22	0
Gooseberries	19	3 heaped tbsp	3	trace	medium
Gooseberries, canned in syrup	73	3 heaped tbsp	18	trace	medium
Gooseberries, stewed	16	3 heaped tbsp	2	trace	medium
Gooseberries, stewed with sugar	54	3 heaped tbsp	13	trace	medium
Gooseberry fool	183	1 serving	20	9	medium
Gooseberry pie	314	1 slice	40	16	medium
Gooseberry sauce	42	1 tbsp	trace	4	medium
Gorgonzola cheese	106	1 small wedge	trace	10	0
Gouda cheese	94	1 small wedge	trace	8	0
Gougère, cheese	239	1 serving	8	24	low
Goulash, hungarian	406	1 serving	16	22	medium

Food	kC/portion	Portion size	Carbs g	Fat g	Fibre
Graham crackers See Digestive biscuits					
Grainy mustard	7	1 tsp	1	trace	low
Granary bread	94	1 medium slice	18	1	medium
Grand marnier	78	1 single measure	7	0	0
Granda padano cheese	113	1 small wedge	trace	8	0
Granola, dry	89	25 g/1 oz/¼ cup	17	1	high
Granola, with semi-skimmed milk	236	3 heaped tbsp	40	5	high
Granola, with skimmed milk	226	3 heaped tbsp	40	3	high
Grape juice	92	1 tumbler	23	trace	0
Grape juice, red	92	1 tumbler	23	trace	0
Grape juice, red, sparkling	61	1 wine glass	16	0	0
Grape juice, white	92	1 tumbler	23	trace	0
Grape juice, white, sparkling	61	1 wine glass	16	0	0
Grapefruit	48	1 fruit	12	trace	medium
Grapefruit, canned in natural juice	30	3 heaped tbsp	7	trace	low
Grapefruit, canned in syrup	60	3 heaped tbsp	15	trace	low
Grapefruit, with port	47	½ grapefruit	8	trace	medium
Grapefruit, with sugar	64	½ grapefruit	16	trace	medium
Grapefruit, with sugar, grilled (broiled)	64	½ grapefruit	16	trace	medium

Food	kC/ portion	Portion size	Carbs g	Fat g	Fibre
Grapefruit cocktail	72	1 serving	18	trace	low
Grapefruit drink, sparkling	88	1 tumbler	24	0	0
Grapefruit juice	66	1 tumbler	17	trace	low
Grapefruit juice drink	72	1 tumbler	18	trace	low
Grapenuts, dry	86	25 g/1 oz/½ cup	20	trace	medium
Grapenuts, with semi-skimmed milk	195	3 heaped tbsp	26	2	medium
Grapenuts, with skimmed milk	183	3 heaped tbsp	26	trace	medium
Grapes, black	60	1 small bunch	15	trace	low
Grapes, green	60	1 small bunch	15	trace	low
Grappa	79	1 single measure	6	0	0
Gravlax	336	1 serving	4	21	0
Gravy, made with giblets or meat juices	56	5 tbsp	2	4	low
Gravy, made with granules	25	5 tbsp	2	2	low
Gravy, thin	2	5 tbsp	trace	trace	0
Greek pastries	322	1 piece	40	17	medium
Greek slow-roasted lamb See Kleftiko					
Greek pork stew See Afelia					
Greek village salad	108	1 serving	5	8	high
Greek-style yoghurt, cows'	161	1 individual pot	5	13	0

Food	kC/ portion	Portion size	Carbs g	Fat g	Fibre
Greek-style yoghurt, sheep's	149	1 individual pot	8	10	0
Greek-style yoghurt, with honey	158	1 serving	15	9	0
Green beans See French (green) beans					
Green chartreuse	78	1 single measure	7	0	0
Green salad	14	1 serving	2	trace	medium
Green salad, dressed	111	1 serving	2	17	medium
Greengage	13	1 fruit	2	trace	medium
Greengage pie	290	1 slice	39	14	medium
Greengages, canned in natural juice	51	3 heaped tbsp	11	trace	medium
Greengages, canned in syrup	69	3 heaped tbsp	16	trace	medium
Greengages, stewed	37	3 heaped tbsp	6	trace	medium
Greengages, stewed with sugar	117	3 heaped tbsp	19	trace	medium
Grenadine syrup, undiluted	35	1 tbsp	9	0	0
Griddle scones (biscuits)	44	1 scone	6	2	low
Grillsteak, minced (ground) beef, grilled (broiled)	185	1 steak	8	12	low
Grillsteak, minced lamb, grilled (broiled)	175	1 steak	1	13	0
Ground beef See Beef, minced					

Food	kC/ portion	Portion size	Carbs g	Fat g	Fibre
Ground rice pudding, made with semi-skimmed milk	205	1 serving	40	11	low
Ground rice pudding, made with skimmed milk	186	1 serving	40	trace	low
Grouper, grilled (broiled)	238	1 piece of fillet	6	3	0
Grouse, roast	456	1 small bird	0	14	0
Gruyère (swiss) cheese	117	1 small wedge	trace	9	0
Guacamole	408	1 serving	1	45	medium
Guard of honour, stuffed	550	2 lamb cutlets	10	42	low
Guava	26	1 medium fruit	5	trace	high
Guava, canned in natural juice	48	3 heaped tbsp	11	0	high
Guava, canned in syrup	60	3 heaped tbsp	16	0	high
Guinea fowl, roast	480	¼ bird	0	14	0
Guinness	117	1 small	6	trace	0

Food	kC/ portion	Portion size	Carbs g	Fat g	Fibre

Food	kC/ portion	Portion size	Carbs g	Fat g	Fibre
Haddock, fried (sautéed), in batter	490	1 piece of fillet	19	26	low
Haddock, fried, in breadcrumbs	435	1 piece of fillet	9	26	low
Haddock, poached or steamed	171	1 piece of fillet	0	1	0
Haddock, smoked, poached	176	1 piece of fillet	0	1	0
Haggis	310	1 serving	19	22	low
Hake, fried (sautéed), in batter	497	1 piece of fillet	19	26	0
Hake, poached or steamed	164	1 piece of fillet2	0	7	0
Halibut, grilled (broiled)	231	1 piece of fillet	0	7	0
Halibut, poached or steamed	229	1 piece of fillet	0	7	0
Halloumi cheese	98	1 thick slice (⅛ block)	1	7	0
Halva	265	¼ block	23	16	low
Ham, boiled	167	2 thick slices	0	5	0
Ham, canned	60	1 medium slice	0	2	0
Ham, ready-sliced, no added water	37	1 medium slice	trace	1	0
Ham, roast	174	2 thick slices	4	6	low
Ham and cheese quiche	476	1 slice	24	32	low
Ham and chopped pork loaf	35	1 slice	trace	3	low
Ham and mushroom pizza, deep-pan	292	1 slice	35	11	medium

Food	kCl/portion	Portion size	Carbs g	Fat g	Fibre
Ham and mushroom pizza, thin-crust	**242**	1 slice	26	9	medium
Ham and pineapple pizza, deep-pan	**276**	1 slice	31	11	medium
Ham and pineapple pizza, thin-crust	**226**	1 slice	22	9	medium
Ham and tomato quiche	**479**	**1 slice**	**25**	**32**	**low**
Ham sandwiches	**341**	1 round	34	18	medium
Hamburger, retail	**253**	1 burger in a bun	33	8	medium
Hamburger, home-made	**437**	1 thick burger in a bun	25	14	low
Hare, jugged	**420**	1 serving	7	30	low
Hare, roast	**193**	1 serving	0	9	0
Hare, stewed	**192**	1 serving	0	8	0
Haricot (navy) beans, canned, drained	**92**	3 heaped tbsp	17	trace	high
Haricot beans, dried, soaked and cooked	**95**	3 heaped tbsp	17	trace	high
Haricot mutton/lamb	**252**	1 serving	24	9	medium
Harusami noodles	**251**	1 serving	57	trace	low
Hash browns	**138**	1 serving	16	8	medium
Haslet	**30**	1 slice	2	2	low
Havarti cheese	**100**	1 slice	0	9	0
Hawaiian pizza, deep-pan	**276**	1 slice	31	11	medium

Food	kC/ portion	Portion size	Carbs g	Fat g	Fibre
Hawaiian pizza, thin-crust	226	1 slice	22	9	medium
Hazelnut (filbert) ice cream	91	1 scoop	12	4	low
Hazelnuts, shelled	162	25 g/1 oz/¼ cup	1	16	high
Hearts, braised	190	1 serving	8	8	high
Hearts, roast, stuffed	295	1 serving	4	19	low
Hearts, stewed	179	1 serving	0	6	0
Herring, grilled (broiled)	202	1 medium fish	0	13	0
Herring, filleted, fried (sautéed), in oatmeal	351	1 medium fish	2	22	low
Herring, pickled	39	1 small fillet	1	3	0
Herring, rollmop	180	1 roll	6	12	0
Herring, soused	180	1 roll	6	12	0
Herring roes, fried (sautéed)	244	1 serving	5	16	low
Herring roes, on toast	399	1 serving plus 1 slice of toast	23	25	low
Hobnobs	69	1 biscuit (cookie)	9	3	low
Hobnobs, chocolate	96	1 biscuit	12	5	low
Hobnob creams, chocolate or vanilla	63	1 biscuit	8	3	low
Hoisin sauce	27	1 tbsp	6	trace	low
Hollandaise sauce	214	3 tbsp	trace	25	0
Homewheat biscuits (cookies), chocolate	87	1 biscuit	11	4	low

Food	kC/portion	Portion size	Carbs g	Fat g	Fibre
Homewheat biscuits, chocolate, mini	**18**	1 biscuit	2	1	low
Honey	**43**	1 tbsp	13	0	0
Honey cake	**89**	1 slice	14	0	low
Honey crispix, dry	**95**	25 g/1 oz/½ cup	21	trace	low
Honey crispix, with semi-skimmed milk	**209**	5 heaped tbsp	33	3	low
Honey crispix, with skimmed milk	**193**	5 heaped tbsp	33	1	low
Honey loops, dry	**92**	25 g/1 oz/½ cup	19	1	medium
Honey loops, with semi-skimmed milk	**205**	5 heaped tbsp	37	3	medium
Honey loops, with skimmed milk	**189**	5 heaped tbsp	37	1	medium
Honey mustard	**7**	1 tsp	trace	trace	0
Honey nut cheerios, dry	**93**	25 g/1 oz/½ cup	20	1	medium
Honey nut cheerios, with semi-skimmed milk	**172**	5 heaped tbsp	30	3	medium
Honey nut cheerios, with skimmed milk	**156**	5 heaped tbsp	30	1	medium
Honey nut corn flakes, dry	**97**	25 g/1 oz/½ cup	20	1	low
Honey nut corn flakes, with semi-skimmed milk	**213**	5 heaped tbsp	39	3	low

Food	kC/ portion	Portion size	Carbs g	Fat g	Fibre
Honey nut corn flakes, with skimmed milk	197	5 heaped tbsp	39	1	low
Honey nut shredded wheat, dry	95	25 g/1 oz/½ cup	17	2	high
Honey nut shredded wheat, with semi-skimmed milk	210	3 heaped tbsp	34	5	high
Honey nut shredded wheat, with skimmed milk	194	3 heaped tbsp	34	3	high
Honey rice krispies, dry	35	25 g/1 oz/½ cup	22	trace	low
Honey rice krispies, with semi-skimmed milk	209	5 heaped tbsp	42	2	low
Honey rice krispies, with skimmed milk	193	5 heaped tbsp	42	trace	low
Honeycomb	42	1 tbsp	11	1	0
Honeydew melon	63	1 large wedge	15	trace	medium
Horlicks, made with semi-skimmed milk	202	1 mug	32	5	low
Horlicks, made with skimmed milk	170	1 mug	32	1	low
Horlicks, instant, chocolate, made with water	128	1 mug	21	3	medium
Horlicks, instant, chocolate malted, made with water	129	1 mug	24	2	medium
Horlicks, instant, low-fat, made with water	127	1 mug	25	1	low

Food	kC/ portion	Portion size	Carbs g	Fat g	Fibre
Horn of plenty mushrooms, fried (sautéed)	78	2 tbsp	trace	8	low
Horn of plenty mushrooms, stewed	6	2 tbsp	trace	trace	low
Horseradish, cream	11	1 tsp	1	1	low
Horseradish, fresh, grated	24	1 tbsp	1	1	low
Horseradish, relish	5	1 tsp	trace	trace	low
Horseradish, sauce	8	1 tsp	1	trace	low
Hot and sour soup	129	2 ladlefuls	8	6	low
Hot chocolate See Drinking (sweetened) chocolate					
Hot cross bun	148	1 bun	26	4	medium
Hot cross bun, with butter	222	1 bun	26	12	medium
Hot cross bun, with low–fat spread	187	1 bun	26	8	medium
Hot dog	189	1 sausage plus 1 bun	22	9	medium
Hot dog, sausage only	82	1 sausage	1	7	low
Hot dog, with onions	230	1 sausage plus 1 bun	4	10	medium
Hot fudge sundae	180	1 sundae30	5	0	
Hummus	280	2 tbsp	13	22	high
Hula hoops See Potato hoops					
Hungarian goulash	406	1 serving8	16	22	medium

Food	kC/ portion	Portion size	Carbs g	Fat g	Fibre
Ice cream, dairy, flavoured	**89**	1 scoop	11	4	low
Ice cream, dairy, vanilla	**97**	1 scoop	12	5	low
Ice cream, low–calorie, flavoured	**67**	1 scoop	8	3	low
Ice cream, low-calorie, vanilla	**71**	1 scoop	9	3	low
Ice cream, mixed, multi-flavours	**91**	1 scoop	12	4	low
Ice cream, non-dairy, flavoured	**83**	1 scoop	11	4	low
Ice cream, non-dairy, vanilla	**89**	1 scoop	11	4	low
Ice cream 99, with flake bar	**175**	1 cornet	31	13	low
Ice cream bombe	**283**	1 serving	18	17	0
Ice cream cone, double	**222**	2 scoops	34	8	low
Ice cream cone, single	**131**	1 scoop	22	4	low
Ice cream gâteau	**227**	1 slice	23	14	low
Ice lolly, any flavour	**28**	1 lolly	7	trace	0
Ice pop, large	**63**	1 lolly	17	0	0
Ice pop, small	**42**	1 lolly	11	0	0
Ice split, any flavour	**83** (avge)	1 lolly	13	3	0
Iceberg lettuce	**2**	1 good handful	1	0	low
Iced coffee	**133**	1 tumbler	10	8	0
Iced coffee, with sugar	**173**	1 tumbler	15	8	0

Food	kC/ portion	Portion size	Carbs g	Fat g	Fibre
Iced (frosted) fancies	150	1 cake	25	5	low
Iced gems	117	1 small bag	25	1	low
Iced tea, with sugar	89	1 tumbler	20	0	0
Icing (frosting) *See individual types and flavours, e.g.* Fondant icing					
Instant whipped dessert, made with semi-skimmed milk	103	1 serving	14	6	low
Instant whipped dessert, made with skimmed milk	88	1 serving	14	3	low
Instant whipped dessert, sugar-free, made with semi-skimmed milk	103	1 serving	11	7	0
Instant whipped dessert, sugar-free, made with skimmed milk	88	1 serving	11	6	0
Irish coffee	218	1 wine glass	7	14	0
Irish cream liqueur	102	1 single measure	6	5	0
Irish stew	336	1 serving	25	21	medium
Irn-bru	65	1 tumbler	21	trace	low
Irn-bru, diet	8	1 tumbler	2	trace	low
Isotonic drink	92	1 can/carton	21	0	0
Italian pork sausage	216	1 sausage	1	17	0

Food	kC/ portion	Portion size	Carbs g	Fat g	Fibre
Jacket potato See also Potato, baked	272	1 large potato	64	trace	high
Jaffa cake	48	1 individual cake	9	1	low
Jaffa cake, mini	26	1 small cake	5	1	low
Jaffa cake muffin	416	1 bar	57	19	low
Jalousie, jam (conserve)	319	1 slice	33	20	low
Jalousie, mincemeat	321	1 slice	33	21	medium
Jam (conserve), any flavour	39	1 tbsp	10	0	0
Jam, any flavour, reduced-sugar	18	1 tbsp	5	trace	0
Jam (jelly) roll), steamed or baked	391	1 slice	52	19	medium
Jam ring biscuits (cookies)	60	1 biscuit	9	2	low
Jam sandwich cake	302	1 slice	64	5	low
Jam sandwich creams	74	1 biscuit (cookie)	9	3	low
Jam sponge cake	302	1 slice	64	5	low
Jam tart	130	1 individual tart	20	5	low
Jambalaya	468	1 serving	61	6	high
Japanese miso soup	78	2 ladlefuls	8	4	medium
Jarlsberg cheese	105	1 small wedge	1	8	0
Jasmine rice	248	1 serving	56	2	low
Jellied consommé	32	2 ladlefuls	2	trace	0

Food	kC/ portion	Portion size	Carbs g	Fat g	Fibre
Jellied eels	70	1 small serving	trace	6	0
Jello See Jelly					
Jelly (jello), any flavour	91	1 serving	22	0	0
Jelly, milk, made with semi-skimmed milk	148	1 serving	28	2	0
Jelly, milk, made with skimmed milk	132	1 serving	28	trace	0
Jelly, sugar-free, made up	8	1 serving	trace	trace	0
Jelly, yoghurt	60	1 serving	12	1	0
Jelly babies	15	1 sweet (candy)	3	0	0
Jelly beans	11	1 bean	3	0	0
Jelly roll See Jam roll *and* Swiss roll					
Jelly tots	147	1 small packet	37	0	0
Jerk chicken	256	1 serving	15	8	high
Jerusalem artichokes, steamed or boiled	41	3 heaped tbsp	11	0	high
Jugged hare	420	1 serving	7	30	low
Jumbo shrimp See King prawn					
Junket, made with semi-skimmed milk	120	1 serving	16	4	0

Food	kC/ portion	Portion size	Carbs g	Fat g	Fibre
Junket, made with skimmed milk	**101**	1 serving	16	2	0
Just right, dry	**90**	25 g/1 oz/½ cup	19	1	medium
Just right, with semi-skimmed milk	**201**	5 heaped tbsp	37	3	medium
Just right, with skimmed milk	**185**	5 heaped tbsp	37	1	medium

Food	kCl/portion	Portion size	Carbs g	Fat g	Fibre
Kalamares, fried (sautéed), in batter	235	1 serving	19	12	low
Kale, steamed or boiled	24	3 heaped tbsp	1	1	medium
Kateifi	322	1 pastry	40	17	medium
Kedgeree, made with smoked fish	498	1 serving	31	24	low
Kedgeree, made with white fish	495	1 serving	31	24	low
Kelp	4	2 tbsp	1	trace	low
Kentucky fried chicken	390	2 pieces	10	27	low
Ketchup (catsup)	15	1 tbsp	4	trace	low
Kettle chips, all flavours	136 (avge)	1 good handful	12	9	medium
Kidney beans See Red kidney beans					
Kidneys, devilled	158	1 serving	2	7	0
Kidneys, lambs', fried (sautéed)	155	2 kidneys	0	6	0
Kidneys, lambs', grilled (broiled)	109	2 kidneys	0	4	0
Kidneys, ox, stewed	172	1 serving	0	8	0
Kidneys, pigs', fried (sautéed)	155	1 kidney	0	6	0
Kidneys, pigs', stewed	153	1 kidney	0	6	0

Food	kC/ portion	Portion size	Carbs g	Fat g	Fibre
Kidneys turbigo	363	1 serving	2	54	low
Kielbasa sausage, grilled (broiled)	81	1 slice	1	7	0
King cone	186	1 cone	29	7	low
King prawn (jumbo shrimp)	10	1 prawn	0	trace	0
King prawn, battered	45	1 prawn	3	2	low
King prawn, in garlic butter	48	1 prawn	trace	2	low
King prawn masala	164	1 serving	5	6	low
Kipper, grilled (broiled)	166	1 medium fish	0	9	0
Kipper, poached or jugged	166	1 medium fish	0	9	0
Kipper fillets, boil-in-the-bag	201	1 fillet	0	15	0
Kipper fillets, canned in oil, drained	140	1 fillet	trace	12	0
Kipper pâté	190	1 serving	trace	17	0
Kir	131	1 wine glass	8	0	0
Kirsch	50	1 single measure	trace	0	0
Kit kat chocolate bar	107	2 fingers	13	5	low
Kit kat chocolate bar, chunky	282	1 bar	33	15	low
Kiwi fruit	46	1 fruit	11	trace	medium
Kleftiko (Greek slow-roast lamb with potatoes)	741	1 serving	11	49	medium
Knackwurst/knockwurst	209	1 sausage	1	19	0

Food	kC/ portion	Portion size	Carbs g	Fat g	Fibre
Knickerbocker glory	**273**	**1 tall glass**	**41**	**10**	**low**
Kohlrabi, steamed or boiled	36	3 heaped tbsp	5	0	medium
Krackawheat	**38**	**1 cracker**	**5**	**2**	**low**
Krispen, all flavours	15 (avge)	1 cracker	3	trace	low
Kulfi ice cream	**340**	**1 serving**	**9**	**32**	**low**
Kumquat	12	1 fruit	3	0	low

Food	kC/ portion	Portion size	Carbs g	Fat g	Fibre
Ladies' fingers See Okra					
Lady fingers See Boudoir					
Lager	**87**	1 small	3	0	0
Lager, high-strength	226	1 small	7	0	0
Lager, low-alcohol	70	1 small	4	0	0
Lamb, breast, roast	**410**	2 thick slices	0	37	0
Lamb, chop, lean, fried (sautéed)	277	1 chop	0	25	0
Lamb, chop, lean, grilled (broiled)	250	1 chop	0	23	0
Lamb, crown roast	488	2 cutlets	0	40	0
Lamb, cutlet, lean, fried	267	1 cutlet	0	22	0
Lamb, cutlet, lean, grilled	244	1 cutlet	0	20	0
Lamb, grillsteak, grilled	175	1 steak	1	13	0
Lamb, guard of honour	550	2 cutlets	10	42	low
Lamb, leg, roast, lean and fat	266	2 thick slices	0	18	0
Lamb, leg, roast, lean only	191	2 thick slices	0	8	0
Lamb, minced (ground), stewed	354	1 serving	0	22	0
Lamb, noisettes, fried	245	2 noisettes	0	14	0
Lamb, noisettes, grilled	222	2 noisettes	0	12	0
Lamb, shank, slow-roasted	465	1 shank	0	31	0

Food	kC/ portion	Portion size	Carbs g	Fat g	Fibre
Lamb, shoulder, roast, lean and fat	316	3 medium slices	0	26	0
Lamb, shoulder, roast, lean only	196	3 medium slices	0	11	0
Lamb, steak, fried (sautéed)	357	1 steak	0	16	0
Lamb, steak, grilled (broiled)	334	1 steak	0	14	0
Lamb byriani	828	1 serving	75	51	medium
Lamb curry	935	1 serving	10	82	medium
Lamb curry, with rice	1183	1 serving	66	84	medium
Lamb goulash	446	1 serving	16	26	medium
Lamb kheema	656	1 serving	5	58	low
Lamb rogan josh	691	1 serving	17	41	medium
Lamb stew	369	1 serving	30	13	medium
Lamb tagine	724	1 serving	14	54	medium
Lambrusco	70	1 wine glass	2	0	0
Lamingtons	233	1 individual cake	36	2	medium
Lancashire cheese	93	1 small wedge	trace	8	0
Lancashire hot-pot	342	1 serving	30	13	high
Langoustines	10	1 langoustine	0	trace	0
Langues de chat	28	1 biscuit (cookie)	3	1	low
Lasagne, meat, home-made	650	1 serving	32	44	medium
Lasagne, meat, ready-prepared	306	1 serving	38	11	low

Food	kC/ portion	Portion size	Carbs g	Fat g	Fibre
Lasagne, seafood	351	1 serving	32	16	high
Lasagne, vegetable	424	1 serving	50	10	high
Lassi	124	1 tumbler	26	trace	low
Leek	44	1 medium leek	6	1	high
Leek, roast	67	1 medium leek	3	3	high
Leek, sliced, steamed or boiled	21	3 heaped tbsp	3	1	medium
Leek and potato soup, canned	94	2 ladlefuls	8	6	low
Leek and potato soup, home-made	117	2 ladlefuls	15	5	medium
Leek and potato soup, packet	80	2 ladlefuls	24	7	low
Leek vinaigrette	223	4 small leeks	3	23	medium
Leerdammer cheese	93	1 small wedge	trace	8	0
Lemon	12	1 fruit	2	trace	0
Lemon and lime, sparkling	78	1 tumbler	19	trace	0
Lemon and lime, sparkling, low-calorie	9	1 tumbler	2	trace	0
Lemon barley water, diluted	40	1 tumbler	9	trace	0
Lemon cake	384	1 slice	54	18	low
Lemon cheesecake	273	1 serving	30	13	low
Lemon chicken	356	1 serving	3	13	0
Lemon curd	42	1 tbsp	9	1	low

Food	kC/ portion	Portion size	Carbs g	Fat g	Fibre
Lemon curd tart	**150**	1 individual tart	22	6	low
Lemon danish pastry	**263**	1 pastry	34	13	medium
Lemon drop cakes	**130**	1 individual cake	20	5	low
Lemon drop sweets (candies)	**20**	1 sweet	5	0	0
Lemon juice, pure	**1**	1 tbsp	trace	trace	low
Lemon meringue pie	**362**	1 slice	50	16	low
Lemon mousse	**227**	1 serving	38	8	low
Lemon puffs	**69**	1 biscuit (cookie)	7	4	low
Lemon sauce	**43**	2 tbsp	10	0	0
Lemon sherbet sweets (candies)	**20**	1 sweet	5	0	0
Lemon slice	**125**	1 cake	19	5	low
Lemon sole, fried (sautéed), in breadcrumbs	**342**	1 medium fish	15	21	low
Lemon sole, grilled (broiled)	**158**	1 medium fish	0	4	0
Lemon sole, poached or steamed	**128**	1 medium fish	0	1	0
Lemon sorbet	**65**	1 scoop	17	trace	0
Lemon soufflé	**315**	1 serving	21	41	0
Lemon sponge pudding	**308**	1 serving	50	11	low
Lemon squash, diluted	**53**	1 tumbler	13	trace	0
Lemon squash, low-calorie, diluted	**2**	1 tumbler	trace	0	0

Food	kC/ portion	Portion size	Carbs g	Fat g	Fibre
Lemon tango	**98**	1 tumbler	23	trace	0
Lemon tango, low-calorie	**8**	1 tumbler	trace	trace	0
Lemon tea, instant	**88**	1 cup	22	0	0
Lemon tea, instant, low-calorie	**5**	1 cup	1	trace	0
Lemon water ice	**65**	1 scoop	17	trace	0
Lemonade, home-made	**141**	1 tumbler	35	trace	0
Lemonade, sparkling	**42**	1 tumbler	11	0	0
Lemonade, sparkling, low-calorie	**1**	1 tumbler	trace	0	0
Lemonade shandy	**60**	1 tumbler	14	trace	low
Lentil and bacon soup, canned	**120**	2 ladlefuls	15	2	medium
Lentil and bacon soup, home-made	**302**	2 ladlefuls4	26	51	medium
Lentil and tomato soup, canned	**108**	2 ladlefuls	20	trace	medium
Lentil rissoles	**90**	1 rissole	15	3	high
Lentil soup, canned	**92**	2 ladlefuls	25	8	medium
Lentil soup, home-made	**198**	2 ladlefuls	26	8	medium
Lentil stew	**282**	1 serving	49	2	high
Lentils, green or brown, soaked and cooked	**105**	3 heaped tbsp	17	1	high

Food	kC/ portion	Portion size	Carbs g	Fat g	Fibre
Lentils, red, cooked	100	3 heaped tbsp	17	trace	medium
Lettuce	2	1 good handful	1	0	low
Lettuce soup, rich, home-made	127	2 ladefuls	19	3	low
Light corn syrup See Golden syrup					
Lilt, pineapple and grapefruit	90	1 tumbler	23	0	0
Lilt, pineapple and grapefruit, diet	8	1 tumbler	0	0	0
Lima beans See Butter beans					
Limburger cheese	93	1 small wedge	trace	8	0
Lime	9	1 fruit	1	0	0
Lime cordial, diluted	36	1 tumbler	10	trace	0
Lime pickle	23	1 tbsp	2	2	low
Lime squash, low-calorie, diluted	2	1 tumbler	trace	0	0
Limeade	16	1 tumbler	4	0	0
Limeade and lager	54	1 tumbler	13	trace	0
Lincoln biscuits (cookies)	43	1 biscuit	6	2	low
Lincolnshire sausage, grilled (broiled)	117	1 sausage	3	9	low
Ling, grilled (broiled)	168	1 piece of fillet	0	1	0

Food	kCl/portion	Portion size	Carbs g	Fat g	Fibre
Linguine (pasta ribbons), dried, boiled	**239**	1 serving	51	2	medium
Linguine, fresh, boiled	**301**	1 serving	57	2	medium
Lion bar, chocolate	**145**	1 standard bar	20	6	low
Lion bar, ice cream	**227**	1 standard bar	24	13	low
Liqueur coffee	**218**	1 wine glass	7	14	0
Liquorice all-sorts	**29**	1 sweet (candy)	7	trace	0
Liquorice caramels	**39**	1 sweet (candy)	7	1	0
Liquorice sticks	**5**	1 stick	1	0	0
Liver, calves', braised	**165**	3 thin slices	3	7	low
Liver, calves', fried (sautéed), in seasoned flour	**254**	3 thin slices	7	13	0
Liver, lambs', fried (sautéed), in seasoned flour	**232**	3 thin slices	4	14	0
Liver, pigs', stewed	**189**	1 serving	4	8	0
Liver and bacon, fried (sautéed)	**498**	1 serving	8	46	0
Liver and onions, fried (sautéed)	**396**	1 serving	18	25	medium
Liver casserole	**220**	1 serving	2	9	low
Liver pâté	**158**	1 serving	trace	14	0
Liver pâté, en croûte	**596**	1 slice	24	49	low

Food	kC/ portion	Portion size	Carbs g	Fat g	Fibre

L

Food	kC/portion	Portion size	Carbs g	Fat g	Fibre
M&Ms, chocolate	219	1 small bag	31	1	0
M&Ms, peanut	231	1 small bag	26	12	low
Macadamia nuts	112	1 small handfu	1	12	high
Macaroni, dried, boiled	198	1 serving	42	1	medium
Macaroni, fresh, boiled	235	1 serving	45	1	medium
Macaroni cheese	436	1 serving	46	17	medium
Macaroni cheese, canned	188	1 small can	19	10	low
Macaroons, almond	120	1 macaroon	13	7	medium
Macaroons, coconut	117	1 macaroon	16	5	medium
Macedoine (mixed, diced vegetables), steamed or boiled	42	3 heaped tbsp	7	trace	high
Mackerel, fried (sautéed)	310	1 medium fish	0	19	0
Mackerel, grilled (broiled)	279	1 medium fish	0	15	0
Mackerel, smoked	531	1 fillet	0	46	0
Mackerel, smoked pâté	599	1 serving	0	58	0
Mackerel, soused	165	1 roll	6	9	0
Madeira, dry	58	1 double measure	trace	0	0
Madeira, sweet	68	1 double measure	trace	0	0
Madeira cake	393	1 slice	58	17	low
Madelaines	137	1 cake	16	8	low
Magnum, all flavours	300 (avge)	1 ice cream	27	20	0

Food	kCl portion	Portion size	Carbs g	Fat g	Fibre
Maids of honour	**207**	1 individual tart	35	12	low
Maître d'hôtel butter	**92**	1 tbsp	trace	10	0
Malt loaf	**80**	1 slice	17	1	low
Maltesers	**183**	1 small packet	18	5	0
Mandarin orange	**30**	1 fruit	7	trace	medium
Mandarin oranges, canned in natural juice	**32**	3 heaped tbsp	8	trace	low
Mandarin oranges, canned in syrup	**52**	3 heaped tbsp	13	trace	low
Mangetout (snow peas)	**16**	3 heaped tbsp	2	trace	medium
Mangetout, steamed or boiled	**13**	3 heaped tbsp	2	trace	medium
Mangetout, stir-fried	**35**	3 heaped tbsp	2	2	medium
Mango	**97**	1 medium fruit	24	trace	high
Mango, canned in syrup	**77**	3 heaped tbsp	20	trace	high
Mango chutney	**43**	1 tbsp	7	2	low
Mango mousse	**137**	1 serving	18	6	low
Mango sorbet	**88**	1 scoop	24	trace	medium
Mangosteen	**20**	1 fruit	5	trace	medium
Mangosteen, canned in syrup	**73**	3 heaped tbsp	18	trace	medium
Maple syrup	**53**	1 tbsp	15	0	0
Maraschino cherries	**12**	1 fruit	3	trace	low
Maraschino liqueur	**64**	1 single measure	8	0	0

Food	kCl portion	Portion size	Carbs g	Fat g	Fibre
Marble cake	371	1 slice	55	14	medium
Marc	55	1 single measure	trace	0	0
Margarine	185	25 g/1 oz/2 tbsp	trace	20	0
Margarine	74	1 small knob	trace	8	0
Margherita pizza, Italian-style	235	1 slice	25	12	medium
Marie biscuits (cookies)	35	1 biscuit	6	1	low
Marlin steak, fried (sautéed)	294	1 steak	0	14	0
Marlin steak, grilled (broiled)	271	1 steak	0	9	0
Marmalade	39	1 tbsp	10	0	low
Marmalade, reduced-sugar	21	1 tbsp	5	trace	0
Marmalade pudding	340	1 serving	45	16	medium
Marmalade tart	285	1 slice	46	11	medium
Marmite	9	1 tsp	trace	trace	0
Marrow (squash), steamed or boiled	9	3 heaped tbsp	2	trace	low
Marrow, stuffed with meat	306	1 large slice	38	8	low
Marrowfat peas, canned	100	3 heaped tbsp	17	1	high
Marrowfat peas, soaked and boiled	82	3 heaped tbsp	18	1	high
Mars chocolate bar	294	1 standard bar	45	11	0
Mars ice cream	209	1 standard bar	22	12	0

Food	kCl/portion	Portion size	Carbs g	Fat g	Fibre
Marsala	**79**	1 double measure	6	0	0
Mascarpone cheese	**128**	1 heaped tbsp	trace	14	0
Marshmallows	**15**	1 sweet (candy)	4	0	0
Marshmallow chocolate tea cakes	**73**	1 cake	13	2	low
Martini, dry	**59**	1 double measure	3	0	0
Martini, sweet	**75**	1 double measure	8	0	0
Marzipan	**101**	25 g/1 oz	17	4	medium
Matchmakers	**10**	1 stick	1	trace	0
Matzos	**100**	1 cracker	23	trace	medium
Mayonnaise	**104**	1 tbsp	trace	11	0
Mayonnaise, low-calorie	**40**	1 tbsp	1	4	0
Mcchicken sandwich	**375**	1 sandwich	39	17	high
Meat and potato pie	**330**	1 serving	25	19	medium
Meat cobbler	**489**	1 serving	40	28	high
Meat paste	**35**	1 tbsp	2	3	low
Meat pie	**460**	1 individual pie	32	28	low
Meatballs, fried (sautéed)	**246**	4 meatballs	0	15	low
Meatballs, grilled (broiled)	**218**	4 meatballs	0	12	0
Meatballs in gravy, canned	**208**	½ large can	9	14	low
Meatballs in tomato sauce, canned	**227**	½ large can	33	7	medium

Food	kCl/ portion	Portion size	Carbs g	Fat g	Fibre
Meatballs with spaghetti	**718**	1 serving	80	31	medium
Meatloaf	**208**	1 thick slice	10	9	low
Meatloaf, with tomato sauce	**370**	2 slices	22	18	medium
Mediterranean vegetables, roasted	**80**	1 serving	10	5	high
Melba toast	**53**	1 slice	11	trace	low
Melon See *individual varieties,* e.g. Cantaloupe melon					
Melon cocktail	**48**	1 serving	12	trace	low
Melon with parma ham	**105**	1 slice of melon plus 2 slices of ham	15	1	low
Melton mowbray pork pie	**677**	1 standard pie	45	48	medium
Meringue	**95**	1 meringue	24	trace	0
Meringue, with cream	**162**	1 meringue	24	7	0
Meringue nest, with fresh fruit	**141**	1 meringue	32	1	medium
Milk loaf	**60**	1 medium slice	12	1	low
Milk powder, dried (non–fat dried milk)	**52**	1 tbsp	8	trace	0
Milk, channel island	**234**	300 ml/½ pt/1¼ cups	14	15	0
Milk, condensed, skimmed, sweetened	**267**	100 ml/3½ fl oz/ scant ½ cup	60	trace	0

Food	kC/ portion	Portion size	Carbs g	Fat g	Fibre
Milk, condensed, whole, sweetened	**333**	100 ml/3½ fl oz/ scant ½ cup	55	10	0
Milk, condensed, skimmed, unsweetened (evaporated)	**80**	100 ml/3½ fl oz/ scant ½ cup	11	trace	0
Milk, condensed, whole, unsweetened (evaporated)	**151**	100 ml/3½ fl oz/ scant ½ cup	8	9	0
Milk, semi-skimmed	**138**	300 ml/½ pt/1¼ cups	15	5	0
Milk, skimmed	**99**	300 ml/½ pt/1¼ cups	15	trace	0
Milk, whole	**198**	300 ml/½ pt/1¼ cups	14	12	0
Milk chocolate	**255**	1 standard bar	28	14	0
Milk classico ice lolly	**141**	1 lolly	9	13	0
Milk jelly (jello), made with semi-skimmed milk	**148**	1 serving	28	2	0
Milk jelly, made with skimmed milk	**132**	1 serving	28	trace	0
Milkshake, extra-thick	**238**	1 tumbler	42	5	low
Milkshake, made with granules and semi-skimmed milk	**138**	1 tumbler	23	3	low
Milkshake, made with granules and skimmed milk	**109**	1 tumbler	23	trace	low
Milkshake, made with syrup and semi-skimmed milk	**125**	1 tumbler	18	3	low

Food	kC/ portion	Portion size	Carbs g	Fat g	Fibre
Milkshake, made with syrup and skimmed milk	**106**	1 tumbler	18	trace	low
Milk stick	**275**	1 lolly	24	18	0
Milky bar chocolate bar	**163**	1 standard bar	17	9	0
Milky way chocolate bar	**117**	1 standard bar	19	4	0
Milky way crispy rolls	**131**	1 roll	14	7	low
Millet flakes	**80**	25 g/1 oz/¼ cup	19	trace	medium
Mince *See individual meats, e.g. Beef, minced*					
Mince pie, sweet	**244**	1 individual pie	39	9	low
Mincemeat	**41**	1 tbsp	9	1	low
Minestrone, canned	**85**	2 ladlefuls	15	1	medium
Minestrone, home–made	**248**	2 ladlefuls	39	7	high
Minestrone, packet	**79**	2 ladlefuls	15	2	medium
Minibix with chocolate, dry	**96**	25 g/1 oz/½ cup	18	1	medium
Minibix with chocolate, with semi-skimmed milk	**212**	3 heaped tbsp	35	4	medium
Minibix with chocolate, with skimmed milk	**196**	3 heaped tbsp	35	3	medium
Minstrels	**206**	1 small packet	29	9	0
Mint chocolate chip ice cream	**91**	1 scoop	12	4	low

Food	kCl/ portion	Portion size	Carbs g	Fat g	Fibre
Mint imperials	**18**	1 sweet (candy)	5	0	0
Mint jelly (clear conserve)	**38**	1 tbsp	6	trace	0
Mint sauce	**18**	1 tbsp	4	trace	0
Miso soup, Japanese	**78**	1 serving	8	4	medium
Mississippi mud pie	**325**	1 slice	38	18	low
Mivi ice lolly, all flavours	**83** (avge)	1 lolly	13	3	0
Mixed (candied) peel	**35**	1 tbsp	9	trace	low
Mixed salad	**31**	1 serving	5	1	high
Mixed salad, dressed	**128**	1 serving	5	18	high
Molasses	**38**	1 tbsp	10	0	0
Monkey nuts, raw, shelled See *also* Peanuts	**85**	1 small handful	2	7	high
Monkfish, grilled (broiled)	**170**	1 piece of fillet	0	3	0
Monkfish, roasted	**216**	1 piece of fillet	0	7	low
Monkfish stew	**330**	1 serving	43	5	medium
Monterey Jack cheese	**106**	1 small wedge	trace	9	0
Morning rolls	**140**	1 roll	29	2	low
Mortadella	**47**	1 slice	trace	4	0
Moules à la crème	**372**	1 serving	11	21	low
Moules à la marinière	**238**	1 serving	11	7	low

Food	kC/ portion	Portion size	Carbs g	Fat g	Fibre
Moussaka	552	1 serving	21	41	medium
Mozzarella cheese, danish	77	1 thick slice (⅛ block)	trace	5	0
Mozzarella cheese, italian	80	¼ round cheese	1	6	0
Muesli, dry	91	25 g/1 oz/¼ cup	16	2	high
Muesli, with semi-skimmed milk	203	3 heaped tbsp	33	5	high
Muesli, with skimmed milk	189	3 heaped tbsp	33	3	high
Muffin, american	169	1 muffin	24	6	medium
Muffin, english	127	1 muffin	25	1	medium
Muffin, english, toasted, with butter	200	1 muffin	25	8	medium
Muffin, english, toasted, with low-fat spread	166	1 muffin	25	5	medium
Mulberries	43	3 heaped tbsp	10	trace	medium
Mulled wine	105	1 wine glass	5	0	0
Mullet, grey or red, grilled (broiled)	139	1 fillet	0	4	0
Mulligatawny soup, canned	137	2 ladlefuls	13	7	medium
Multi-grain start, dry	90	25 g/1 oz/½ cup	20	trace	medium
Multi-grain start, with semi-skimmed milk	201	5 heaped tbsp	38	3	medium
Multi-grain start, with skimmed milk	185	5 heaped tbsp	38	1	medium

Food	kCl portion	Portion size	Carbs g	Fat g	Fibre
Munchies	22	1 sweet	3	1	0
Mung beans, dried, soaked and cooked	**105**	3 heaped tbsp	18	trace	high
Mung beans, sprouted	**6**	1 good handful	1	trace	high
Mung beans, sprouted, canned	**12**	3 heaped tbsp	2	trace	high
Munster cheese	**104**	1 small wedge	trace	8	0
Muscatels, stoned (pitted)	**41**	1 small handful	10	trace	low
Mushroom bhaji	**123**	1 bhaji	9	8	medium
Mushroom ketchup	**6**	1 tsp	trace	trace	0
Mushroom omelette	**295**	2 eggs	trace	26	low
Mushroom pâté	**117**	½ small tub	4	9	0
Mushroom pâté, home-made	**191**	1 serving	1	19	low
Mushroom and cheese quiche	**353**	1 slice	18	26	low
Mushroom ragu	**311**	1 serving	3	30	low
Mushroom risotto	**341**	1 serving	52	14	low
Mushroom pasta sauce	**45**	¼ jar	7	10	0
Mushroom sauce, made with semi-skimmed milk	**99**	5 tbsp	8	6	low
Mushroom sauce, made with skimmed milk	**89**	5 tbsp	8	5	low
Mushroom soup, cream of, canned	**106**	2 ladlefuls	8	8	0

Food	kCl/portion	Portion size	Carbs g	Fat g	Fibre
Mushroom soup, home-made	**156**	2 ladlefuls	14	2	low
Mushroom soup, low-fat, canned	**48**	2 ladlefuls	7	1	low
Mushroom soup, packet	**118**	2 ladlefuls	21	2	0
Mushroom soup, instant	**96**	1 mug	13	5	0
Mushrooms _See also individual types, e.g. Shiitake mushrooms_	**2**	1 medium mushroom	trace	trace	low
Mushrooms, breaded	**196**	1 serving	8	16	low
Mushrooms, button, sliced and fried (sautéed)	**78**	1 serving	trace	8	low
Mushrooms, large, flat, fried	**157**	2 large mushrooms	trace	16	low
Mushrooms, stewed	**5**	3 heaped tbsp	trace	trace	low
Mushrooms, stuffed	**53**	1 large mushroom	4	2	low
Mushrooms à la grecque	**171**	1 serving	4	30	low
Mushy peas, canned	**69**	3 heaped tbsp	16	trace	high
Mussels, cooked, shelled	**3**	1 mussel	trace	trace	0
Mussels, smoked, canned, drained	**96**	½ small can	2	5	0
See also Moules					
Mustard _See individual varieties, e.g. Dijon mustard_					

Food	kC/ portion	Portion size	Carbs g	Fat g	Fibre
Mustard and cress	2	1 tbsp	trace	medium	
Mustard butter	118	1 tbsp	trace	6	0
Mustard chicken	176	1 breast	3	5	0
Mustard sauce, made with semi-skimmed milk	103	5 tbsp	6	low	
Mustard sauce, made with skimmed milk	93	5 tbsp	8	5	low
Mutton, boiled	253	2 thick slices	0	16	0
Mutton, haricot	252	1 serving	24	9	medium
Mutton pie	225	1 individual pie	24	5	medium
Mutton stew	369	1 serving	24	21	medium

Food	kC/ portion	Portion size	Carbs g	Fat g	Fibre
Naan bread, plain	175	1 small bread	29	4	medium
Nachos with cheese	346	6 pieces	36	19	low
Napoletana pizza	247	1 slice	25	13	medium
Napoletana sauce	61	¼ jar	9	2	low
Navy beans *See Haricot beans*					
Neapolitan ice cream	86	1 scoop	10	4	0
Nectarine	52	1 fruit	12	trace	medium
Nesquick cereal, dry	98	25 g/1 oz/½ cup	21	1	low
Nesquick cereal, with semi-skimmed milk	179	5 heaped tbsp	31	3	low
Nesquick cereal, with skimmed milk	163	5 heaped tbsp	31	1	low
Nesquick milk shake flavouring *See Milkshakes*					
Neufchatel cheese	74	1 small wedge	1	7	0
Nice biscuits (cookies)	35	1 biscuit	5	1	low
Niçoise salad	308	1 serving	34	11	high
Noilly prat	59	1 double measure	3	0	0
Noisettes of lamb, grilled (broiled)	222	2 noisettes	0	12	0
Noodles, dried, boiled	239	1 serving	51	2	medium

Food	kC/ portion	Portion size	Carbs g	Fat g	Fibre
Noodles, fresh, boiled	**301**	1 serving	57	2	medium
See also individual types, e.g. Chinese egg noodles					
Norwegian apple cake	**252**	1 slice	32	10	high
Norwegian blue cheese	**87**	1 small wedge	trace	7	0
Norwegian cream	**835**	1 serving	25	79	0
Nut brittle	**226**	1 standard bar	34	9	medium
Nut cutlet	**139**	1 cutlet	5	10	medium
Nut rissole	**203**	1 rissole	6	18	medium
Nut roast	**366**	1 serving	13	29	high
Nutri-grain breakfast bars, all flavours	**130** (avge)	1 bar	24	3	medium
Nuts See individual varieties, e.g. brazil nuts					
Nuts, mixed	**151**	25 g/1 oz/¼ cup	2	13	high
Nuts and raisins	**108**	1 small handful	7	7	high

Food	kCl/portion	Portion size	Carbs g	Fat g	Fibre
Oat bran	51	1 tbsp	9	1	high
Oat bran crispbread	27	1 crispbread	5	trace	medium
Oat bran flakes, dry	87	25 g/1 oz/½ cup	16	1	high
Oat bran flakes, with semi-skimmed milk	197	5 heaped tbsp	33	4	high
Oat bran flakes, with skimmed milk	181	5 heaped tbsp	33	2	high
Oat cereal, instant See Ready brek					
Oat flakes, dry	96	25 g/1 oz/½ cup	17	18	high
Oat flakes, with semi-skimmed milk	211	5 heaped tbsp	33	5	high
Oat flakes, with skimmed milk	195	5 heaped tbsp	33	3	high
Oat krunchies, dry	98	25 g/1 oz/¼ cup	19	1	medium
Oat krunchies, with semi-skimmed milk	214	5 heaped tbsp	25	3	medium
Oat krunchies, with skimmed milk	198	5 heaped tbsp	25	1	medium
Oatcakes	59	1 oatcake	8	2	medium
Oatmeal	94	25 g/1 oz/¼ cup	16	2	medium
Oatmeal porridge, made with semi-skimmed milk	207	1 serving	32	6	medium

Food	kC/ portion	Portion size	Carbs g	Fat g	Fibre
Oatmeal porridge, made with skimmed milk	191	1 serving	32	6	medium
Oatmeal porridge, made with water	150	1 serving	26	4	medium
Oats, rolled	100	25 g/1 oz/¼ cup	18	1	medium
Oats, rolled, porridge, made with semi-skimmed milk	217	1 serving	35	6	medium
Oats, rolled, porridge, made with skimmed milk	201	1 serving	35	4	medium
Oats, rolled, porridge, made with water	160	1 serving	29	4	medium
Octopus	164	1 serving	4	2	0
Octopus, marinated in olive oil	200	½ small can	2	16	0
Ogen melon	57	½ melon	13	trace	medium
Oil, all types	135	1 tbsp	0	15	0
Okra (ladies' fingers), steamed or boiled	28	3 heaped tbsp	3	1	high
Okra, stir-fried	269	3 heaped tbsp	4	26	high
Olives, black or green	7	1 olive	trace	trace	medium
Olives, stuffed	4	1 olive	trace	trace	medium
Olives, with feta cheese	19	1 piece of each	trace	2	low

Food	kCl/ portion	Portion size	Carbs g	Fat g	Fibre
Omelette See also individual fillings, e.g. Cheese omelette	256	2 eggs	trace	22	0
Omelette arnold bennet	373	2 eggs	trace	29	0
Onion	36	1 medium onion	8	trace	medium
Onion, fried (sautéed)	82	2 tbsp	7	5	medium
Onion, pickled	4	1 onion	1	trace	low
Onion, spring (scallion)	3	1 onion	trace	trace	low
Onion, stuffed	190	1 large onion	19	8	high
Onion bhaji	123	1 bhaji	9	8	medium
Onion dip	27	2 tbsp	1	1	0
Onion pakoras	148	1 pakora	9	11	medium
Onion rings, deep-fried in batter or breadcrumbs	97	5 rings	9	6	low
Onion sauce, made with semi-skimmed milk	64	5 tbsp	6	4	low
Onion sauce, made with skimmed milk	55	5 tbsp	6	3	low
Onion soup, cream of, canned	88	2 ladlefuls	8	6	low
Onion soup, french, home-made	94	2 ladlefuls	8	6	low
Onion soup, french, packet	104	2 ladlefuls	20	1	low

Food	kC/ portion	Portion size	Carbs g	Fat g	Fibre
Onion soup, french, with cheese croûte	226	2 ladlefuls plus 1 croûte	21	8	low
Onion soup, white, home-made	121	2 ladlefuls	12	3	low
Onion soup, white, packet	77	2 ladlefuls	4	trace	low
Onions in white sauce	36	3 heaped tbsp	6	1	high
Orange	57	1 fruit	13	1	medium
Orange and pineapple pure fruit juice	84	1 tumbler	22	trace	low
Orange and pineapple squash, diluted	96	1 tumbler	22	trace	0
Orange and pineapple squash, low-calorie, diluted	22	1 tumbler	5	trace	0
Orange barley water, diluted	40	1 tumbler	10	trace	0
Orange cake	290	1 slice	32	17	low
Orange curd	42	1 tbsp	9	1	low
Orange ice lolly	78	1 lolly	19	0	0
Orange jelly (jello), fresh	40	1 serving	7	0	low
Orange mousse	137	1 serving	18	6	low
Orange pure fruit juice	72	1 tumbler	14	trace	low
Orange sauce	40	2 tbsp	10	trace	0
Orange squash, diluted	96	1 tumbler	22	trace	0

Food	kC/portion	Portion size	Carbs g	Fat g	Fibre
Orange squash, low-calorie, diluted	24	1 tumbler	5	trace	0
Orange tango	92	1 tumbler	25	0	0
Orange tango, low-calorie	9	1 tumbler	2	trace	0
Orange water ice	64	1 scoop	16	0	0
Orangeade, sparkling	20	1 tumbler	4	0	0
Oranges in caramel	139	1 serving	33	1	medium
Original crunchy cereal, dry	97	25 g/1 oz/¼ cup	16	3	high
Original crunchy cereal, with semi-skimmed milk	250	3 heaped tbsp	37	7	high
Original crunchy cereal, with skimmed milk	234	3 heaped tbsp	37	5	high
Osso buco	382	1 serving	17	10	low
Ovaltine, made with semi-skimmed milk	197	1 mug	32	4	low
Ovaltine, made with skimmed milk	165	1 mug	32	trace	low
Ovaltine light, instant, made with water	72	1 mug	13	1	low
Oven chips (fries) See Chips					
Ox tongue, sliced	73	1 slice	0	6	0
Oxo	27	1 cube	4	trace	0

Food	kCl/portion	Portion size	Carbs g	Fat g	Fibre
Oxo drink	**10**	1 mug	trace	0	0
Oxtail soup, canned	**88**	2 ladlefuls	10	3	0
Oxtail soup, packet	**54**	2 ladlefuls	8	2	0
Oxtail soup, instant	**77**	1 mug	14	2	0
Oxtail and vegetable stew	**318**	1 serving	7	15	high
Oyster mushrooms	**1**	1 mushroom	trace	trace	low
Oyster mushrooms, fried (sautéed)	**77**	2 tbsp	trace	8	low
Oyster mushrooms, stewed	**3**	2 tbsp	trace	trace	low
Oysters	**7**	1 oyster	trace	trace	0
Oysters, fried (sautéed), in batter	**368**	6 oysters	40	18	low
Oysters, smoked, canned, drained	**103**	½ small can	trace	6	0

Food	kC/ portion	Portion size	Carbs g	Fat g	Fibre
Paella, dried	294	1 serving	55	3	low
Paella, home-made	411	1 serving	34	11	low
Pain au chocolat	236	1 pastry	26	13	low
Pain au raisin	212	1 pastry	27	10	medium
Pain perdu	213	1 slice	17	18	low
Pak choi/soi	19	1 head	2	trace	medium
Pak choi/soi, steamed or boiled	12	3 heaped tbsp	2	trace	medium
Pak choi/soi, stir-fried	36	3 heaped tbsp	2	2	medium
Pakora	148	1 pakora	9	11	medium
Palm hearts, canned, drained	9	1 piece	2	trace	low
Palmiers	83	1 piece	12	6	low
Pancake, buckwheat	45	1 pancake	6	2	low
Pancake, potato	207	1 pancake	22	11	medium
Pancake, scotch	44	1 pancake	6	2	low
Pancake, wheat	100	1 pancake	8	6	low
See also Crêpe and Drop scone					
Pancake, with lemon and sugar	120	1 pancake	13	6	low
Pancake roll, large	217	1 large roll	21	12	low
Pancake roll, small	70	1 small roll	7	3	low
Pancetta, diced, fried (sautéed)	248	2 tbsp	0	22	0

Food	kC/ portion	Portion size	Carbs g	Fat g	Fibre
Panna cotta	328	1 serving	38	17	low
Pappardelle (pasta ribbons), dried, boiled	239	1 serving	51	2	medium
Pappardelle, fresh, boiled	301	1 serving	57	2	medium
Papaya	118	1 fruit	30	trace	high
Papaya, canned in natural juice	65	3 heaped tbsp	17	trace	low
Paratha	450	1 paratha	62	20	high
Parkin	185	1 piece	29	7	low
Parma ham	21	1 slice	0	1	0
Parma ham, with figs	87	1 fig plus 2 slices of ham	11	2	medium
Parma ham, with melon	105	1 slice of melon plus 2 slices of ham	15	1	low
Parmesan cheese	113	1 small chunk	trace	8	0
Parmesan cheese, grated	68	1 tbsp	trace	5	0
Parsley sauce, made with semi-skimmed milk	99	5 tbsp	8	6	low
Parsley sauce, made with skimmed milk	89	5 tbsp	8	5	low
Parsnips	112	1 medium parsnip	22	2	high
Parsnips, roasted	156	4 pieces	22	6	high
Parsnips, steamed or boiled	66	1 serving	13	1	high
Partridge, roast	212	½ small bird	0	7	0

Food	kC/ portion	Portion size	Carbs g	Fat g	Fibre
Passata (sieved tomatoes)	29	5 tbsp	6	trace	0
Passion fruit	17	1 fruit	4	trace	medium
Passion fruit ice cream	83	1 scoop	11	3	0
Pasta salad	197	1 serving	28	8	high
Pasta sauce, traditional, ready-made _See also individual flavours, e.g._ Tomato and herb	58	¼ jar	8	2	0
Pasta, shapes, dried, boiled	198	1 serving	42	1	medium
Pasta shapes, fresh, boiled	235	1 serving	45	2	medium
Pasta shapes, wholemeal, dried, boiled	218	1 serving	44	2	high
Pasta strands, all sizes, dried, boiled	239	1 serving	51	2	medium
Pasta strands, fresh, boiled	301	1 serving	57	2	medium
Pasta strands, wholemeal, dried, boiled	259	1 serving	152	6	high
Pastis	61	1 single measure	trace	0	0
Pastrami	99	1 slice	1	8	0
Pastrami, on rye bread	154	1 slice of each	12	8	medium
Pâté, with toast and butter	496	1 serving plus 2 slices of toast	35	31	medium

Food	kC/ portion	Portion size	Carbs g	Fat g	Fibre
Pavlova, topped with cream and fruit	**320**	1 serving	45	14	medium
Paw paw	**118**	1 fruit	30	trace	high
Pea and ham soup, canned	**150**	2 ladlefuls	19	6	high
Pea and ham soup, packet	**150**	2 ladlefuls	18	7	medium
Pea soup, canned	**188**	2 ladlefuls	30	6	medium
Pea soup, instant	**95**	1 mug	16	2	medium
Peach	**42**	1 peach	11	trace	medium
Peach and apple pure fruit juice	**84**	1 tumbler	20	trace	low
Peach melba	**169**	1 serving	28	5	medium
Peach pie	**261**	1 slice	38	12	low
Peach chutney	**24**	1 tbsp	6	trace	low
Peach squash, diluted	**96**	1 tumbler	22	trace	0
Peach squash, low-calorie, diluted	**24**	1 tumbler	5	trace	0
Peaches, dried	**31**	1 piece	8	trace	high
Peaches, dried, stewed with sugar	**103**	3 heaped tbsp	27	trace	high
Peaches, dried, stewed	**77**	3 heaped tbsp	20	trace	high
Peaches, sliced, canned in natural juice	**39**	3 heaped tbsp	10	trace	low

Food	kC/portion	Portion size	Carbs g	Fat g	Fibre
Peaches, sliced, canned in syrup	55	3 heaped tbsp	14	trace	low
Peaches, whole, poached in natural juice	80	1 peach	16	trace	medium
Peaches, whole, poached in syrup	101	1 peach	16	trace	medium
Peaches, whole, poached in wine	136	1 peach	17	trace	medium
Peanut brittle	226	1 standard bar	34	9	medium
Peanut butter	93	1 tbsp	2	8	high
Peanut butter and chocolate spread	89	1 tbsp	5	7	medium
Peanut cookies	116	1 cookie	13	6	high
Peanut sauce	220	5 tbsp	8	18	medium
Peanuts, dry-roasted	88	1 small handful	1	7	medium
Peanuts, raw, shelled	141	25 g/1 oz/¼ cup	3	11	medium
Peanuts, roasted, salted	90	1 small handful	1	8	medium
Peanuts and raisins	70	1 small handful	5	5	medium
Pear	45	1 fruit, unpeeled	11	trace	high
Pear and apple pure fruit juice	78	1 tumbler	20	0	0
Pear condé	356	1 serving	51	15	medium

Food	kC/portion	Portion size	Carbs g	Fat g	Fibre
Pear drops	**16**	1 sweet (candy)	4	0	0
Pear melba	**179**	1 serving	32	5	low
Pearl barley, cooked	**101**	1 serving	23	trace	medium
Pears, canned in natural juice	**70**	2 halves	17	trace	medium
Pears, canned in syrup	**100**	2 halves	25	trace	medium
Pears, dried	**47**	1 piece	12	trace	high
Pears, dried, stewed	**127**	3 heaped tbsp	34	trace	high
Pears, dried, stewed with sugar	**140**	3 heaped tbsp	37	trace	high
Pears, poached in wine	**139**	1 pear	7	trace	medium
Pears with chocolate sauce	**348**	1 serving	87	2	high
Peas, dried, soaked and boiled	**109**	3 heaped tbsp	20	1	high
Peas, fresh, shelled	**83**	3 heaped tbsp	11	1	high
Peas, fresh, shelled, cooked	**79**	3 heaped tbsp	10	2	high
Peas, frozen, cooked	**69**	3 heaped tbsp	10	1	high
Peas, garden, canned, drained	**80**	3 heaped tbsp	13	1	high
Peas, garden, canned, drained	**100**	3 heaped tbsp	17		
Peas, marrowfat, soaked and cooked	**82**	3 heaped tbsp	18	1	high
Peas, mushy, canned	**81**	3 heaped tbsp	14	1	medium
Peas, processed, canned, drained	**99**	3 heaped tbsp	17	1	high

Food	kC/ portion	Portion size	Carbs g	Fat g	Fibre
Peas, split, soaked and boiled	262	3 heaped tbsp	20	16	high
Peas, sugar snap	**57**	10 pods	8	1	high
Peas, sugar snap, steamed or boiled	52	3 heaped tbsp	5	1	high
Pease pudding	**109**	3 heaped tbsp	20	1	high
Pecan nuts, shelled	196	25 g/1 oz/¼ cup	2	20	high
Pecan pie	**502**	1 slice	64	27	medium
Pecorino cheese	113	1 small chunk	trace	8	0
Peking duck with pancakes	**665**	1 portion with 6 small pancakes	32	42	high
Penne rigate (pasta shapes), dried, boiled	**198**	1 serving	42	1	medium
Penne rigate, fresh, boiled	235	1 serving	45	2	medium
Penguin chocolate bars, all flavours	**135** (avge)	1 standard bar	17	7	low
Peperami	132	1 stick	trace	12	low
Peppermint cordial, diluted	36	1 tumbler	10	trace	0
Peppermints	18	1 mint	5	0	0
Peperoni	27	1 slice	trace	2	0
Peperoni pizza	255	1 slice	28	10	low
Pepper (bell), green	22	1 pepper	4	trace	medium
Pepper, green, roasted	45	1 pepper	4	5	medium

Food	kC/ portion	Portion size	Carbs g	Fat g	Fibre
Pepper, green, stewed	27	1 pepper	4	1	medium
Pepper, orange/yellow	35	1 pepper	7	trace	medium
Pepper, orange/yellow, roasted	58	1 pepper	7	5	medium
Pepper, orange/yellow, stewed	39	1 pepper	7	1	medium
Pepper, red	48	1 pepper	10	1	medium
Pepper red, roasted	71	1 pepper	10	6	medium
Pepper red, stewed	51	1 pepper	10	1	medium
Pepper, stuffed with meat	266	1 pepper	27	8	medium
Pepper, stuffed with rice	202	1 pepper	36	5	high
Pepsi	88	1 tumbler	22	0	0
Pepsi, diet	0	1 tumbler	trace	0	0
Pepsi max	1	1 tumbler	trace	0	0
Pernod	55	1 single measure	trace	0	0
Perry, sparkling	70	1 wineglass	0	2	0
Persimmon	32	1 fruit	8	trace	low
Pesto sauce	64	1 tbsp	trace	7	low
Petit pois, cooked	49	3 heaped tbsp	17	1	high
Petit suisse cheese	23	1 small pot	1	1	0
Petits fours	23	1 sweet (candy)	3	1	low
Petticoat tails shortbread	64	1 wedge	7	3	low
Pheasant, roast	536	¼ bird	0	24	0

Food	kC/ portion	Portion size	Carbs g	Fat g	Fibre
Pheasant à la normande	675	¼ bird	3	46	low
Pheasant casserole	588	¼ bird	20	30	low
Physalis	3	1 fruit	trace	trace	low
Piccalilli	13	1 tbsp	3	trace	low
Pickle, sweet	20	1 tbsp	5	trace	low
Pickle, tomato	24	1 tbsp	6	trace	low
Pickled egg	84	1 egg	trace	6	0
Pickled onion, large	4	1 onion	1	trace	low
Pickled onion, silverskin	2	1 onion	trace	trace	low
Picnic chocolate bar	230	1 standard bar	29	11	medium
Pigeon, roast	303	½ large or 1 small bird	0	18	0
Pigeon casserole	333	½ large or 1 small bird	8	20	low
Pigeon pie	470	1 serving	21	28	medium
Pike, grilled (broiled)	175	1 piece of fillet	0	1	0
Pikelets	91	1 pikelet	19	trace	low
Pilaff	286	1 serving	45	9	medium
Pilau rice	212	1 serving	46	2	medium
Pilchards, in tomato sauce, canned	177	2 pilchards	3	7	low
Pimientos, canned, drained	21	1 pimiento	8	1	low
Pimms	146	1 tumbler	11	0	0

Food	kC/ portion	Portion size	Carbs g	Fat g	Fibre
Pina colada	**252**	1 cocktail	32	3	low
Pine nuts	**172**	25 g/1 oz/¼ cup	1	17	medium
Pineapple	**41**	1 slice	10	trace	medium
Pineapple, chunks, canned in natural juice	47	3 heaped tbsp	12	trace	low
Pineapple, glacé (candied)	13	1 piece	4	trace	low
Pineapple, with kirsch	132	2 slices	29	trace	medium
Pineapple and grapefruit drink, sparkling	**88**	1 tumbler	24	trace	0
Pineapple and grapefruit pure fruit juice	**94**	1 tumbler	24	0	low
Pineapple and grapefruit squash, diluted	**96**	1 tumbler	22	trace	0
Pineapple and grapefruit squash, low-calorie, diluted	24	1 tumbler	5	trace	0
Pineapple flambé	**122**	1 slice	24	1	medium
Pineapple pure fruit juice	**82**	1 tumbler	21	trace	low
Pineapple sorbet	**65**	1 scoop	17	trace	0
Pineapple upside–down pudding	**367**	1 slice	58	14	medium
Pineapple water ice	**65**	1 scoop	17	trace	0
Pink champagne	**114**	1 wineglass	2	0	0

Food	kC/ portion	Portion size	Carbs g	Fat g	Fibre
Pink gin	**56**	1 cocktail	0	trace	0
Pink grapefruit	**48**	1 fruit	12	trace	medium
Pink grapefruit, with sugar	64	½ fruit	16	trace	medium
Pink grapefruit, with sugar, grilled (broiled)	64	½ fruit	16	trace	medium
Pinto beans, refried	**237**	1 serving	39	3	high
Pinto beans, soaked and boiled	137	3 heaped tbsp	24	1	high
Piperade	**260**	1 serving	18	17	medium
Pistachio nut ice cream	**91**	1 scoop	12	4	low
Pistachio nuts, unshelled	**50**	1 small handful	1	4	high
Pitta bread, party size	**16**	1 tiny bread	4	trace	low
Pitta bread, white	160	1 bread	36	trace	medium
Pitta bread, white, small	80	1 small bread	18	trace	low
Pitta bread, wholemeal	**137**	**1 bread**	**27**	**1**	**high**
Pizza, cheese and tomato, deep-pan	**300**	1 slice	30	14	medium
Pizza, cheese and tomato, thin-crust *See also other flavours, e.g Ham and mushroom pizza*	235	1 slice	25	12	medium
Plaice, grilled (broiled)	**202**	1 medium fish	0	7	0

Food	kCl/portion	Portion size	Carbs g	Fat g	Fibre
Plaice, fillet, fried (sautéed), in batter	**488**	1 fillet	24	31	low
Plaice, fillet, fried (sautéed), in breadcrumbs,	**399**	1 fillet	15	24	low
Plaice, fillet, steamed or poached	**162**	1 fillet	0	3	0
Plantain, boiled or steamed	**112**	½ plantain	28	trace	medium
Plantain, fried (sautéed)	**267**	½ plantain	47	9	medium
Ploughman's lunch	**650**	1 serving	54	36	medium
Plum, large	**30**	1 fruit	7	trace	medium
Plum, small	**11**	1 fruit	2	trace	medium
Plum crumble	**298**	1 serving	51	10	medium
Plum fool	**227**	1 serving	36	8	medium
Plum jam (conserve)	**39**	1 tbsp	10	0	low
Plum pie	**290**	1 slice	14	39	medium
Plum pudding	**291**	1 serving	49	10	medium
Plum sauce, oriental	**27**	1 tbsp	6	trace	low
Plums, canned in syrup	**59**	3 heaped tbsp	15	trace	low
Plums, stewed	**27**	3 heaped tbsp	6	trace	medium
Plums, stewed with sugar	**107**	3 heaped tbsp	19	trace	medium
Poires belle hélène	**348**	1 serving	87	2	high
Polenta (cornmeal)	**214**	1 serving	46	1	low

Food	kC/ portion	Portion size	Carbs g	Fat g	Fibre
Polenta, with cheese	320	1 serving	46	14	low
Polenta, with meat sauce	431	1 serving	51	18	low
Pollack, baked	178	1 piece of fillet	0	2	0
Polish pork sausage	185	¼ ring	1	16	0
Polo mints	120	1 tube	34	trace	0
Polo mints, sugar-free	80	1 tube	33	0	0
Polony	70	1 slice	3	5	0
Pomegranate	51	1 fruit	12	trace	high
Pommes dauphinoise	235	1 serving	12	15	medium
Pompano, grilled (broiled)	186	1 piece of fillet	0	11	0
Pont l'évêque cheese	101	1 small wedge	trace	8	0
Pontefract cakes	8	1 sweet (candy)	2	0	0
Pop tarts, all flavours	202 (avge)	1 tart	36	6	medium
Poppadoms, fried (sautéed)	48	1 poppadom	6	2	low
Poppadoms, grilled (broiled)	35	1 poppadom	6	trace	low
Popcorn, plain	148	1 small handful	16	8	medium
Popcorn, sweet, buttered	122	1 small handful	22	4	medium
Pork, chop, barbecued	210	1 chop	1	9	0
Pork, chop, lean, fried (sautéed)	222	1 chop	0	14	0
Pork, chop, lean, grilled (broiled)	199	1 chop	0	9	0

Food	kC/ portion	Portion size	Carbs g	Fat g	Fibre
Pork, escalope, fried (sautéed)	185	1 escalope	0	7	0
Pork, loin, smoked	56	1 slice	0	3	0
Pork, minced (ground), lean, stewed	147	1 serving	0	7	0
Pork, roast, with crackling	286	2 thick slices	0	20	0
Pork, roast, without crackling	185	2 thick slices	0	7	0
Pork, sweet and sour	303	1 serving	31	9	medium
Pork and beef sausages, thick, fried (sautéed)	115	1 sausage	5	8	low
Pork and beef sausages, thick, grilled (broiled)	111	1 sausage	5	8	low
Pork and beef sausages, thin, fried	57	1 sausage	2	4	low
Pork and beef sausages, thin, grilled	55	1 sausage	2	4	low
Pork and vegetable stir-fry	273	1 serving	18	10	high
Pork belly, grilled (broiled)	398	1 slice	0	35	0
Pork belly, pickled	280	1 slice	0	22	0
Pork chop suey	321	1 serving	34	9	medium
Pork chow mein	323	1 serving	34	8	high
Pork crackling	101	1 finger-sized piece	0	13	0

Food	kC/ portion	Portion size	Carbs g	Fat g	Fibre
Pork kebab, marinated and grilled (broiled)	227	1 kebab	12	10	0
Pork pie	677	1 individual pie	45	49	medium
Pork rillettes	115	2 tbsp	0	10	0
Pork sausages, extra-lean, fried (sautéed)	92	1 sausage	4	5	low
Pork sausages, extra-lean, grilled (broiled)	84	1 sausage	4	5	low
Pork sausages, thick, fried	123	1 sausage	4	10	low
Pork sausages, thick, grilled	117	1 sausage	5	10	low
Pork sausages, thin, fried	61	1 sausage	2	5	low
Pork sausages, thin, grilled	58	1 sausage	2	5	low
Pork spare ribs, barbecued american-style	288	2 ribs	2	16	0
Pork spare ribs, chinese-style	310	2 ribs	13	17	low
Pork teriyaki	133	1 serving	2	5	low
Porridge, instant See Ready brek					
Porridge, made with semi-skimmed milk	217	1 serving	35	6	medium
Porridge, made with skimmed milk	201	1 serving	35	4	medium
Porridge, made with water	160	1 serving	29	4	medium

Food	kC/portion	Portion size	Carbs g	Fat g	Fibre
Port salut cheese	100	1 small wedge	trace	8	0
Port, ruby, tawny or white	78	1 double measure	6	0	0
Pot au chocolat	136	1 individual pot	19	5	low
Pot au chocolat, with cream	270	1 individual pot	20	19	low
Pot noodle, all flavours	305 (avge)	1 pot	42	10	low
Potato, baked in jacket	272	1 large potato	64	trace	high
Potato, baked in jacket, with butter	346	1 large potato	64	8	high
Potato cake	126	1 cake	16	5	low
Potato chips See Crisps					
Potato hoops, all flavours	131 (avge)	1 small packet	14	8	low
Potato pancake	207	1 pancake	22	11	medium
Potato salad, canned	176	3 heaped tbsp	15	10	low
Potato salad, with French dressing	217	3 heaped tbsp	27	11	medium
Potato salad, with mayonnaise, home-made	200	3 heaped tbsp	17	12	medium
Potato waffle, cooked	84	1 waffle	13	3	low
Potato wedges	205	6 wedges	34	4	high

Food	kC/ portion	Portion size	Carbs g	Fat g	Fibre
Potatoes, chipped (fries), home-made	312	1 serving	50	11	high
Potatoes, creamed	104	1 serving	15	4	medium
Potatoes, croquette, shallow-fried	107	1 croquette	11	6	medium
Potatoes, duchesse	82	1 piece	8	2	medium
Potatoes, mashed, instant	57	3 heaped tbsp	13	trace	low
Potatoes, mashed, with butter or margarine	104	3 heaped tbsp	15	4	medium
Potatoes, new, boiled or steamed	75	3 small potatoes	18	trace	medium
Potatoes, new, canned	63	3 small potatoes	15	trace	low
Potatoes, steamed	72	2 pieces	17	trace	medium
Potatoes, roast	149	2 pieces	26	4	medium
Potatoes, scalloped	86	1 serving	11	4	medium
Potted cheese	267	1 small pot	1	23	0
Potted prawns (shrimp)	358	1 small pot	0	32	0
Potted shrimps	324	1 small pot	0	31	0
Poussin (cornish hen), roast, with skin	668	1 bird	0	47	0
Poussin, roast, without skin	295	1 bird	0	8	0

Food	kCl/portion	Portion size	Carbs g	Fat g	Fibre
Poussin, spatchcocked, grilled (broiled)	428	1 bird	0	30	0
Praline ice cream	91	1 scoop	12	4	low
Prawn, king (jumbo shrimp), plain-cooked	10	1 prawn	0	trace	0
Prawn and vegetable stir-fry	250	1 serving	30	5	medium
Prawn and avocado sandwiches	454	1 round	35	30	medium
Prawn and lettuce sandwiches	347	1 round	34	18	medium
Prawn byriani	707	1 serving	75	32	medium
Prawn chop suey	225	1 serving	34	2	medium
Prawn choux balls	79	1 ball	2	8	low
Prawn chow mein	262	1 serving	28	1	high
Prawn cocktail	160	1 serving	4	9	low
Prawn crackers	44	1 small handful	10	1	low
Prawn curry	220	1 serving	36	5	medium
Prawn fajitas	300	2 fajitas	34	13	high
Prawn jalfrezi	465	1 serving	54	9	high
Prawn mayonnaise sandwiches	513	1 round	36	27	medium
Prawn risotto	389	1 serving	84	18	low

Food	kC/ portion	Portion size	Carbs g	Fat g	Fibre
Prawn rogan josh	562	1 serving	17	27	medium
Prawn salad	137	1 serving	5	2	high
Prawn salad, dressed	240	1 serving	5	13	high
Prawn toast	53	1 toast	2	4	low
Prawns (shrimp), canned, drained	80	½ small can	0	1	0
Prawns, cooked, peeled	53	2 tbsp	0	1	0
Prawns in garlic butter	284	1 serving	trace	24	0
Pretzel flipz	235	1 small bag	33	9	low
Pretzels	20	1 small handful	4	trace	low
Prickly pear	42	1 fruit	10	trace	high
Processed cheese slice	65	1 slice	trace	5	0
Profiteroles with chocolate sauce	373	1 serving	33	24	medium
Provolone cheese	99	1 small wedge	1	7	0
Prune juice	136	1 tumbler	36	trace	low
Prunes	11	1 prune	3	trace	high
Prunes, canned in natural juice	79	3 heaped tbsp	20	trace	high
Prunes, canned in syrup	90	3 heaped tbsp	23	trace	high
Ptarmigan, roast	216	1 small or ½ large	0	8	0
Puffed wheat, dry	80	25 g/1 oz/½ cup	17	trace	medium

Food	kC/ portion	Portion size	Carbs g	Fat g	Fibre
Puffed wheat, with semi-skimmed milk	**185**	5 heaped tbsp	33	2	medium
Puffed wheat, with skimmed milk	**169**	5 heaped tbsp	33	trace	medium
Pumpernickel	**93**	1 slice	20	trace	medium
Pumpkin, canned	**34**	3 heaped tbsp	8	trace	medium
Pumpkin, steamed or boiled	**13**	3 heaped tbsp	2	trace	medium
Pumpkin pie	**316**	1 slice	41	14	low
Pumpkin seeds	**81**	1 small handful	3	7	high
Puri	**328**	1 piece	43	25	medium

Food	kC/ portion	Portion size	Carbs g	Fat g	Fibre
Quail, roast	205	1 bird	0	6	0
Quail's eggs, cooked	15	1 egg	trace	1	0
Quality street chocolates	37	1 sweet (candy)	5	2	0
Quark	15	1 tbsp	trace	trace	0
Quarterpounder with cheese	516	1 burger in a bun	37	27	high
Quavers	96	1 small packet	9	6	low
Queen cakes	245	1 individual cake	26	15	low
Queen of puddings	341	1 serving	46	13	low
Queen scallops, poached or steamed	12	4 scallops	0	trace	0
Quenelles, fish	90	1 ball/roll	3	7	0
Quesadillas	225	3 pieces	27	9	high
Quiche anglaise	387	1 slice	17	31	low
Quiche lorraine	476	1 slice	24	32	low
See also individual flavours, e.g. Cheese and onion quiche					
Quince	17	1 fruit	4	trace	low
Quince jelly (clear conserve)	55	1 tbsp	13	trace	0
Quinoa	93	25 g/1 oz/3 tbsp	17	1	medium
Quinoa porridge, made with semi-skimmed milk	206	1 serving	34	4	medium

Food	kC/ portion	Portion size	Carbs g	Fat g	Fibre
Quinoa porridge, made with skimmed milk	190	1 serving	34	2	medium
Quinoa wholegrain cereal	149	1 serving	28	2	medium
Quorn, chunks	74	1 serving	2	3	high
Quorn, fillets	44	1 fillet	2	1	medium
Quorn, fillets, in breadcrumbs	185	1 fillet	13	10	high
Quorn, minced (ground)	79	1 serving	1	3	high
Quorn, sweet and sour	149	1 serving	29	1	medium
Quorn burger	117	1 burger	6	5	high
Quorn cottage pie	212	1 serving	32	6	medium
Quorn fajitas	303	2 fajitas	45	7	high
Quorn sausages	115	1 sausage	5	5	high
Quorn southern burgers	178	1 burger	12	10	high
Quorn spaghetti bolognese	292	1 serving	38	6	high
Quorn tikka masala, with rice	540	1 serving	74	21	high

Food	kC/ portion	Portion size	Carbs g	Fat g	Fibre
Rabbit and vegetable stew	404	1 serving	35	3	high
Radicchio	6	½ head	1	trace	medium
Radish	1	1 radish	trace	trace	low
Radish, winter	12	1 radish	2	trace	low
Rainbow trout, grilled (broiled)	240	1 medium fish	0	10	0
Raisin bread	86	1 slice	15	7	low
Raisin fudge	87	1 square	15	2	low
Raisin wheats, dry	80	25 g/1 oz/½ cup	17	trace	high
Raisin wheats, with semi-skimmed milk	185	3 heaped tbsp	34	3	high
Raisin wheats, with skimmed milk	169	3 heaped tbsp	34	1	high
Raisins, seedless	41	1 small handful	10	trace	high
Raisins, stoned (pitted)	41	1 small handful	11	trace	high
Rambutans	7	1 fruit	2	trace	low
Rambutans canned in syrup	82	3 heaped tbsp	21	trace	low
Raspberries	25	3 heaped tbsp	5	trace	medium
Raspberries, canned in natural juice	71	3 heaped tbsp	17	trace	medium
Raspberries, canned in syrup	88	3 heaped tbsp	22	trace	medium
Raspberries, stewed	20	3 heaped tbsp	4	trace	medium
Raspberries, stewed with sugar	48	3 heaped tbsp	11	trace	medium

Food	kCl/portion	Portion size	Carbs g	Fat g	Fibre
Raspberry jam (conserve)	39	1 tbsp	10	0	0
Raspberry milkshake, made with granules See *also* Milkshake	138	1 tumbler	23	3	low
Raspberry mousse	137	1 serving	18	6	low
Raspberry pavlova	320	1 serving	45	14	medium
Raspberry ripple ice cream	96	1 scoop	12	4	0
Raspberry sauce	28	2 tbsp	7	trace	medium
Raspberry sorbet	57	1 scoop	19	trace	low
Raspberry soufflé	315	1 serving	21	41	0
Raspberry tart	271	1 slice	24	18	low
Ratafia biscuits (cookies)	21	1 biscuit	4	trace	low
Ratatouille	191	3 heaped tbsp	11	15	high
Ravioli, dried, boiled	291	1 serving	45	6	medium
Ravioli, fresh, boiled	248	1 serving	32	8	medium
Ravioli, in beef and tomato sauce, canned	154	½ large can	23	5	medium
Ravioli, in tomato sauce, canned	140	½ large can	20	4	medium
Ray See Skate					
Ready-to-roll icing (frosting)	96	25 g/1 oz	23	0	0
Ready brek, dry	89	25 g/1 oz/½ cup	15	2	medium

Food	kC/ portion	Portion size	Carbs g	Fat g	Fibre
Ready brek, with semi-skimmed milk	210	5 heaped tbsp	31	6	high
Ready brek, with skimmed milk	191	5 heaped tbsp	31	3	high
Ready brek, chocolate, dry	90	25 g/1 oz/½ cup	16	2	medium
Ready brek, chocolate, with skimmed milk	199	5 heaped tbsp	33	3	high
Ready brek, chocolate, with semi-skimmed milk	215	5 heaped tbsp	33	5	high
Real fruit winders, all flavours	55 (avge)	1 roll	11	1	low
Red beet See Beetroot					
Red bull	45	1 can	11	0	0
Red kidney beans, canned, drained	100	3 heaped tbsp	18	1	high
Red kidney beans, dried, soaked and cooked	103	3 heaped tbsp	17	trace	high
Red leicester cheese	101	1 small wedge	trace	8	0
Red salmon See Salmon					
Red snapper, baked, stuffed	146	1 medium fish	12	2	low
Red snapper, grilled (broiled)	218	1 medium fish	0	3	0
Red windsor cheese	100	1 small wedge	trace	8	0
Red wine sauce	63	5 tbsp	9	2	0

Food	kC/ portion	Portion size	Carbs g	Fat g	Fibre
Redcurrant jelly (clear conserve)	55	1 tbsp	13	trace	0
Redcurrants	28	3 heaped tbsp	7	trace	high
Redcurrants, frosted	27	1 small bunch	7	trace	high
Refried beans	237	1 serving	39	3	high
Revels	173	1 small packet	23	6	0
Rhubarb, canned in syrup	31	3 heaped tbsp	8	trace	low
Rhubarb, stewed	7	3 heaped tbsp	1	trace	medium
Rhubarb, stewed with sugar	48	3 heaped tbsp	11	trace	medium
Rhubarb crumble	297	1 serving	51	10	medium
Rhubarb fool	237	1 serving	38	8	medium
Rhubarb pie	290	1 slice	14	39	medium
Rhubarb sauce	137	2 tbsp	34	trace	medium
Ribena, diluted	103	1 tumbler	27	0	0
Rice, long-grain, boiled	248	1 serving	56	2	low
Rice, brown, boiled	254	1 serving	58	2	medium
Rice, fried (sautéed) See *also* Egg fried rice *and* Special fried rice	236	1 serving	45	6	medium
Rice, savoury	256	1 serving	47	6	medium
Rice and peas	247	1 serving	53	3	high
Rice cakes	35	1 individual cake	7	trace	low
Rice drink	100	1 tumbler	20	trace	0

Food	kC/portion	Portion size	Carbs g	Fat g	Fibre
Rice, jasmine	248	1 serving	56	2	low
Rice krispies, dry	92	25 g/1 oz/½ cup	21	trace	low
Rice krispies, with semi-skimmed milk	205	5 heaped tbsp	40	2	low
Rice krispies, with skimmed milk	189	5 heaped tbsp	40	trace	low
Rice milk	150	300 ml/½ pt/1¼ cups	30	1	0
Rice noodles, boiled	251	1 serving	57	trace	low
Rice pudding, canned	323	½ large can	43	15	low
Rice pudding, canned, low-fat	136	½ large can	23	2	low
Rice pudding, made with semi-skimmed milk	150	1 serving	29	2	low
Rice pudding, made with skimmed milk	134	1 serving	29	trace	low
Rich tea biscuits (cookies)	39	1 biscuit	6	1	low
Ricicles, dry	90	25 g/1 oz/½ cup	22.2	0.2	low
Ricicles, with semi-skimmed milk	201	5 heaped tbsp	15	2	low
Ricicles, with skimmed milk	185	5 heaped tbsp	15	trace	low
Ricotta cheese, made with semi-skimmed milk	38	1 heaped tbsp	trace	2	0
Ricotta cheese, whole milk	42	1 heaped tbsp	trace	4	0
Rigatoni (pasta shapes), dried, boiled	198	1 serving	42	1	medium

Food	kCl/portion	Portion size	Carbs g	Fat g	Fibre
Rigatoni, fresh, boiled	235	1 serving	45	2	medium
Ripple chocolate bar	175	1 standard bar	19	10	0
Risotto *See also individual flavours, e.g. Mushroom risotto*	336	1 serving	52	14	low
Risotto, sprinkled with cheese	449	1 serving	52	22	low
Risotto alla milanese	403	1 serving	58	18	low
Rissoles	134	1 rissole	8	9	low
Ritz original crackers	17	1 cracker	1	1	low
Ritz cheese crackers	17	1 cracker	1	1	low
Ritz cheese sandwich crackers	45	1 sandwich cracker	5	2	low
Riva chocolate bar	136	1 standard bar	14	8	low
Roasted nut cereal bar	181	1 bar	24	8	medium
Rock cakes	176	1 individual cake	27	7	low
Rock salmon, fried (sautéed), in batter	580	1 fillet	21	44	low
Rocket (arugula)	2	1 good handful	trace	trace	medium
Rocky chocolate bars, all flavours	125 (avge)	1 standard bar	15	7	low
Roes *See Cod roes and Herring roes*					
Rollmop herring	180	1 roll	6	12	0

Food	kC/ portion	Portion size	Carbs g	Fat g	Fibre
Rolos	269	1 tube	38	12	0
Romano cheese	110	1 small wedge	1	8	0
Root beer	135	1 tumbler	35	0	0
Roquefort cheese	105	1 small wedge	trace	9	0
Rose hip syrup, undiluted	35	1 tbsp	9	0	0
Roses chocolates	39	1 sweet (candy)	5	2	0
Rosti	156	1 serving	25	5	medium
Rotelli (pasta shapes), dried, boiled	198	1 serving	42	1	medium
Rotelli, fresh, boiled	235	1 serving	45	2	medium
Rouille	151	1 tbsp	2	15	low
Roulade *See individual flavours e.g. Chocolate roulade*					
Roulé, garlic and herb cheese	77	1 good spoonful	1	7	low
Roulé, light	28	1 good spoonful	1	2	0
Royal game soup	88	2 ladlefuls	10	4	low
Royal icing (frosting)	58	1 tbsp	15	0	0
Rum, dark	55	1 single measure	trace	0	0
Rum, white	55	1 single measure	trace	0	0
Rum and black	123	1 single measure	18	0	0
Rum and coke	94	1 single measure plus 1 mixer	6	0	0

Food	kC/ portion	Portion size	Carbs g	Fat g	Fibre
Rum and low-calorie cola	56	1 single measure plus 1 mixer	trace	0	0
Rum and raisin fudge	87	1 square	15	2	0
Rum and raisin ice cream	124	1 scoop	12	4	low
Rum and raisin sauce	145	2 tbsp	32	2	low
Rum baba	326	1 individual cake	47	10	low
Rum butter	73	1 tbsp	8	4	0
Rum punch	116	1 wine glass	15	trace	0
Rum sauce, made with semi-skimmed milk	50	5 tbsp	5	2	low
Rum sauce, made with skimmed milk	47	5 tbsp	5	trace	low
Rump steak See Steak, rump or sirloin					
Runner beans, steamed or boiled	18	3 heaped tbsp	2	trace	medium
Ruote (pasta), dried, boiled	198	1 serving	42	1	medium
Ruote, fresh, boiled	235	1 serving	45	2	medium
Russian salad	62	2 tbsp	5	4	high
Rutabaga See Swede					
Rye bread	55	1 medium slice	11	trace	medium
Rye bread, light	35	1 medium slice	12	trace	medium
Ryvita	27	1 crispbread	5	trace	medium

Food	kC/ portion	Portion size	Carbs g	Fat g	Fibre
Sabayon sauce	43	5 tbsp	4	1	0
Sag aloo	163	1 serving	21	9	high
Sage derby cheese	101	1 small wedge	trace	9	0
Sago pudding, canned	167	½ large can	27	7	low
Sago pudding, made with semi-skimmed milk	150	1 serving	29	2	low
Sago pudding, made with skimmed milk	134	1 serving	29	trace	low
Saint paulin cheese	100	1 small wedge	trace	8	0
Saithe *See Coley*					
Salad cream	52	1 tbsp	2	5	0
Salad cream, reduced-calorie	29	1 tbsp	1	2	0
Salade niçoise	308	1 serving	34	11	high
Salami, hard-cured	41	1 slice	trace	3	0
Salami, moist-cured	57	1 slice	trace	5	0
Salmon, baked, stuffed	199	1 steak	5	8	low
Salmon, canned, drained	155	½ small can	0	4	0
Salmon, grilled (broiled)	367	1 piece of fillet	0	25	0
Salmon, in filo pastry (paste)	495	1 portion	8	17	low
Salmon, poached or steamed	345	1 piece of fillet	0	23	0
Salmon, smoked *See also entries for Smoked salmon*	119	2 thin slices	0	4	0

Food	kCl/portion	Portion size	Carbs g	Fat g	Fibre
Salmon, with hollandaise sauce	559	1 serving	trace	48	0
Salmon and cucumber sandwiches	378	1 round	35	21	medium
Salmon en croûte	757	1 serving	46	54	low
Salmon fish cakes, fried (sautéed)	213	1 cake	15	11	low
Salmon fish cakes, grilled (broiled)	192	1 cake	17	7	low
Salmon mousse	205	1 serving	6	6	low
Salmon paste	33	1 tbsp	trace	2	0
Salmon pâté	308	1 serving	0	28	0
Salmon quiche	363	1 slice	17	25	low
Salmon salad	376	1 serving	5	24	high
Salmon salad, with mayonnaise	582	1 serving	5	47	high
Salmon sandwiches	374	1 round	34	21	medium
Salsa, fresh chilli	18	1 tbsp	4	trace	medium
Salsa, fresh tomato	14	1 tbsp	1	1	medium
Salsify, steamed or boiled	23	3 heaped tbsp	9	trace	high
Saltwater crayfish See Dublin bay prawns					
Sambal	20	2 tbsp	4	1	medium

Food	kC/ portion	Portion size	Carbs g	Fat g	Fibre
Samosa, meat	300	1 samosa	9	28	low
Samosa, vegetable	236	1 samosa	11	21	medium
Sangria	66	1 wine glass	4	0	0
Sardine and tomato paste	23	1 tbsp	trace	1	0
Sardine pâté	238	1 serving	0	24	0
Sardines, canned in oil, drained	108	½ small can	0	7	0
Sardines, canned in tomato sauce	88	½ small can	trace	6	low
Sardines, canned, on toast	263	3 sardines plus 1 slice of toast	8	15	low
Sardines, fresh, grilled (broiled)	67	1 good-sized fish	0	4	0
Satsuma	23	1 fruit	5	trace	medium
Sauerkraut, drained	19	3 heaped tbsp	4	trace	medium
Sausage and bacon rolls	105	1 roll	1	24	low
Sausage and egg mcmuffin	427	1 portion	25	26	medium
Sausage in batter, fried (sautéed)	235	1 sausage	23	15	low
Sausage mcmuffin	360	1 portion	26	23	medium
Sausage roll, cocktail	52	1 small roll	3	1	low
Sausage roll, jumbo	477	1 large roll	22	24	medium

Food	kC/ portion	Portion size	Carbs g	Fat g	Fibre
Sausage roll, puff pastry (paste)	238	1 standard roll	16	18	low
Sausage roll, shortcrust pastry (basic pie crust)	229	1 standard roll	18	16	low
Sausages See individual meats, e.g. Pork sausages					
Savarin	326	1 slice	47	10	low
Saveloy	170	1 sausage	6	13	low
Savoury rice, cooked	109	1 serving	24	0	medium
Scallion See Spring onion					
Scallops, fried (sautéed), in breadcrumbs	32	1 scallop	1	1	low
Scallops, steamed or poached	12	1 scallop	0	trace	0
Scallops mornay	210	1 serving	18	3	low
Scaloppine, fried (sautéed), in breadcrumbs	335	1 scallopine	20	15	low
Scampi, fried (sautéed), in batter	360	8 pieces	24	16	low
Scampi, fried (sautéed), in breadcrumbs	316	8 pieces	29	17	low
Scampi provençal	286	1 serving	9	10	medium
Schloer	61	1 tumbler	16	0	0
Schnapps	55	1 single measure	trace	0	0

Food	kCl portion	Portion size	Carbs g	Fat g	Fibre
Schnitzel, fried (sautéed), in breadcrumbs	335	1 schnitzel	20	15	low
Scone (biscuit)	181	1 scone	27	7	low
Scone, cheese	175	1 scone	21	9	low
Scone, drop (small pancake)	44	1 pancake	6	2	low
Scone, fruit	158	1 scone	26	5	low
Scone, griddle	44	1 scone	6	2	low
Scone, plain, with butter	255	1 scone	27	15	low
Scone, plain, with low-fat spread	220	1 scone	27	11	low
Scone, sweet	201	1 scone	32	7	low
Scone, sweet, with butter	275	1 scone	32	15	low
Scone, sweet, with low-fat spread	240	1 scone	32	11	low
Scone, with clotted cream and jam (conserve)	308	1 scone	37	16	low
Scotch broth, canned	88	2 ladlefuls	14	2	medium
Scotch broth, home-made	156	2 ladlefuls	19	3	high
Scotch egg	301	1 egg	16	20	low
Scotch pancake	44	1 pancake	6	2	low
Scotch pie	225	1 individual pie	24	5	medium
Scotch woodcock	487	1 slice	18	39	low

Food	kC/ portion	Portion size	Carbs g	Fat g	Fibre
Scrambled eggs on toast	**463**	2 eggs plus 1 slice of toast	19	37	low
Sea bass, grilled (broiled)	**153**	1 piece of fillet	0	4	0
Seafood cocktail	**134**	1 cocktail	4	9	low
Seafood enchiladas	**562**	2 enchiladas	78	14	medium
Seafood lasagne	**351**	1 serving	32	16	high
Seafood pasta	**460**	1 serving	62	4	high
Seafood pasta salad	**261**	1 serving	29	5	medium
Seafood pizza, thin-crust	**250**	1 slice	25	13	medium
Seafood pizza, deep-pan	**315**	1 slice	30	15	medium
Seafood salad	**106**	1 serving	5	2	high
Seafood salad, with mayonnaise	**312**	1 serving	5	24	high
Seafood sticks	**12**	1 stick	1	trace	0
Seakale, steamed or boiled	**24**	3 heaped tbsp	1	1	medium
Seaweed	**4**	2 tbsp	1	trace	low
Seaweed, deep-fried	**131**	3 heaped tbsp	3	12	medium
Seed cake	**423**	1 slice	58	20	low
Semolina (cream of wheat), canned	**172**	½ large can	27	5	low
Semolina, made with semi-skimmed milk	**150**	1 serving6	29	2	low

Food	kC/ portion	Portion size	Carbs g	Fat g	Fibre
Semolina, made with skimmed milk	134	1 serving	29	trace	low
Sesame seeds	90	1 tbsp	trace	9	high
Seven-up	88	1 tumbler	22	0	0
Seven-up, diet	3	1 tumbler	0	0	0
Seviche	193	1 serving	3	18	low
Shandy	48	1 tumbler	13	trace	0
Shark steak, fried (sautéed)	283	1 steak	0	13	0
Shark steak, grilled (broiled)	260	1 steak	0	8	0
Shark's fin soup	99	2 ladlefuls	8	7	0
Sheep's milk	285	300 ml/½ pt/1¼ cups	15	18	medium
Shepherd's pie	330	1 serving	25	19	medium
Sherbet dip	78	1 small packet	19	0	0
Sherbet drink	91	1 tumbler	20	1	0
Sherbet fountain	88	1 tube	21	0	0
Sherbet lemons	20	1 sweet (candy)	5	0	0
Sherbet oranges	20	1 sweet (candy)	5	0	0
Sherbet pips	4	1 pip	1	0	0
Sherried chicken	197	¼ small chicken	7	4	low
Sherry, dry (fino)	58	1 double measure	1	0	0
Sherry, medium (amontillado)	59	1 double measure	2	0	0

Food	kC/portion	Portion size	Carbs g	Fat g	Fibre
Sherry, sweet (oloroso)	68	1 double measure	3	0	0
Shiitake mushrooms, fresh, fried (sautéed)	50	2 tbsp	6	5	low
Shiitake mushrooms, fresh, stewed	27	2 tbsp	6	trace	low
Shiitake mushrooms, reconstituted dried, stewed	35	1 tbsp	7	trace	low
Shish kebabs	176	1 kebab	0	8	0
Shortbread fingers	67	1 finger	8	3	low
Shortcake biscuits (cookies)	43	1 biscuit	6	2	low
Shredded wheat, dry	74	1 biscuit	15	trace	high
Shredded wheat, with semi-skimmed milk	205	2 biscuits	36	2	high
Shredded wheat, with skimmed milk	189	2 biscuits	36	1	high
Shredded wheat bitesize, dry	84	25 g/1 oz/½ cup	17	trace	high
Shredded wheat bitesize, with semi-skimmed milk	208	3 heaped tbsp	37	3	high
Shredded wheat bitesize, with skimmed milk	192	3 heaped tbsp	37	1	high
Shreddies, dry	86	25 g/1 oz/½ cup	18	trace	high
Shreddies, with semi-skimmed milk	213	5 heaped tbsp	38	3	high

Food	kC/ portion	Portion size	Carbs g	Fat g	Fibre
Shreddies, with skimmed milk	197	5 heaped tbsp	38	1	high
Shreddies, chocolate, dry	91	25 g/1 oz/½ cup	20	trace	medium
Shreddies, chocolate, with semi-skimmed milk	224	5 heaped tbsp	42	3	high
Shreddies, chocolate, with skimmed milk	208	5 heaped tbsp	42	1	high
Shreddies, frosted, dry	91	25 g/1 oz/½ cup	20	trace	high
Shreddies, frosted, with semi-skimmed milk	224	5 heaped tbsp	43	3	high
Shreddies, frosted, with skimmed milk	208	5 heaped tbsp	43	1	high
Shrimp See Prawns					
Shrimps, canned, drained	80	½ small can	0	trace	0
Shrimps, brown or pink, cooked, peeled	15	2 tbsp	0	trace	0
Shrimps, potted	358	1 small pot	0	32	0
Shropshire blue cheese	87	1 small wedge	trace	7	0
Sieved tomatoes See Passata					
Sild, in oil, drained	108	½ small can	0	7	0
Silverskin onions	2	1 onion	trace	trace	low
Simnel cake	298	1 slice	49	11	medium
Skate wings, in batter	367	1 wing	9	22	low

Food	kC/ portion	Portion size	Carbs g	Fat g	Fibre
Skate wings, in black butter	470	1 wing	trace	41	0
Skippers, in oil, drained	108	½ small can	0	7	0
Skips	87	1 small packet	10	5	low
Slivovitz	55	1 single measure	trace	0	0
Sloe gin	35	1 single measure	8	0	0
Smacks, dry	95	25 g/1 oz/⅓ cup	21	trace	low
Smacks, with semi-skimmed milk	209	5 heaped tbsp	40	3	low
Smacks, with skimmed milk	193	5 heaped tbsp	40	1	low
Smarties (M&Ms)	170	1 tube	26	9	0
Smelts, fried (sautéed), in seasoned flour	525	5 fish	5	47	low
Smoked chicken breast	23	1 slice	trace	1	0
Smoked fish See *individual fish, e.g. Salmon, smoked, also Smoked haddock and Smoked salmon*					
Smoked haddock roulade	377	1 serving	16	20	low
Smoked pork ring	185	¼ ring	1	16	0
Smoked salmon	119	2 thin slices	0	4	0
Smoked salmon sandwiches	363	1 round	34	19	medium
Smoked salmon and cream cheese bagel	353	1 bagel	44	12	medium

Food	kC/ portion	Portion size	Carbs g	Fat g	Fibre
Smoked salmon and cream cheese sandwiches	**429**	1 round	34	26	medium
Smoked salmon pâté	**273**	1 serving	0	26	0
Smoked turkey breast	**21**	1 slice	trace	trace	0
Snack shortcake	**40**	1 biscuit (cookie)	5	2	low
Snack wafer bar	**65**	1 finger	7	4	0
Snails, in garlic butter	**311**	6 snails	trace	25	low
Snapper, grilled (broiled)	**218**	1 medium fish	0	3	0
Snickers chocolate bar	**329**	1 standard bar	36	18	low
Snickers ice cream bar	**230**	1 standard bar	20	15	low
Snow peas See Mangetout					
Soba noodles, cooked	**228**	1 serving	48	trace	high
Soda bread, brown	**80**	1 thick slice	15	2	low
Soda bread, white	**82**	1 thick slice	12	2	low
Softgrain bread See Bread					
Sole *See individual varieties, and cooking methods, e.g. Dover sole, Sole meunière, etc.*					
Sole meunière	**376**	1 medium fish	trace	22	0
Sole mornay	**243**	1 fillet	7	12	low
Sole véronique	**184**	1 fillet	11	6	low
Solero ice lolly	**130**	1 lolly	20	4	0

Food	kCl/portion	Portion size	Carbs g	Fat g	Fibre
Somen noodles, boiled	230	1 serving	48	trace	medium
Soufflé *See individual flavours, e.g. Cheese soufflé*					
Soufflé omelette, savoury	256	2 eggs	trace	22	0
Soufflé omelette, sweet	374	2 eggs	10	22	0
Soupe au pistou, canned	60	2 ladlefuls	13	1	medium
Soured (dairy sour) cream and chive dressing	38	1 tbsp	trace	3	low
Soused herring	180	1 roll	6	12	0
Soused mackerel	165	1 roll	6	9	0
Southern comfort	70	1 single measure	4	0	0
Southern fried chicken	494	2 pieces	19	29	low
Soy sauce	10	1 tsp	1	0	0
Soya beans, canned, drained	140	3 heaped tbsp	5	7	high
Soya beans, dried, soaked and cooked	141	3 heaped tbsp	5	7	high
Soya cheese	106	1 small wedge	trace	9	0
Soya cream substitute	28	1 tbsp	1	3	low
Soya desserts, all flavours	103 (avge)	1 individual pot	19	2	low
Soya ice desserts, all flavours	44 (avge)	1 scoop	5	2	low

Food	kC/ portion	Portion size	Carbs g	Fat g	Fibre
Soya milk, sweetened	120	300 ml/½ pt/1¼ cups	12	5	low
Soya milk, unsweetened	96	300 ml/½ pt/1¼ cups	2	6	low
Soya yoghurt	90	1 individual pot	5	5	low
Spaghetti, dried, boiled	239	1 serving	51	2	medium
Spaghetti, dried, wholemeal, boiled	259	1 serving	152	6	high
Spaghetti, fresh, boiled	301	1 serving	57	2	medium
Spaghetti, with clams	433	1 serving	52	6	medium
Spaghetti, with meatballs	718	1 serving	80	31	medium
Spaghetti, with sausages in tomato sauce, canned	116	1 small can	25	9	medium
Spaghetti, with tomato sauce	432	1 serving	71	13	high
Spaghetti, with tomato sauce, canned	128	1 small can	27	1	medium
Spaghetti, with tomato sauce, no-added-sugar, canned	101	1 small can	20	1	medium
Spaghetti alfredo	478	1 serving	67	13	high
Spaghetti bolognese	456	1 serving	56	19	medium
Spaghetti carbonara	402	1 serving	56	22	medium
Spaghetti hoops, canned	122	1 small can	26	1	medium
Spaghetti hoops with hot dogs, canned	180	1 small can	22	8	low

Food	kCl/portion	Portion size	Carbs g	Fat g	Fibre
Spaghetti napoletana	**432**	1 serving	71	13	high
Spam	**86**	1 slice	trace	8	0
Spanish omelette	**328**	2 eggs	17	22	medium
Spanish rice	**228**	1 serving	46	2	high
Spare ribs See Pork spare ribs					
Special fried rice	**362**	1 serving	54	9	high
Special K, dry	**92**	25 g/1 oz/½ cup	18	trace	low
Special K, with semi-skimmed milk	**205**	5 heaped tbsp	36	trace	low
Special K, with skimmed milk	**189**	5 heaped tbsp	36	trace	low
Special K red berries, dry	**92**	25 g/1 oz/½ cup	18	trace	low
Special K red berries, with semi-skimmed milk	**205**	5 heaped tbsp	36	2	low
Special K red berries, with skimmed milk	**189**	5 heaped tbsp	36	trace	low
Spinach	**12**	1 good handful	1	trace	medium
Spinach, cooked	**19**	3 heaped tbsp	1	1	medium
Spinach, frozen, cooked	**21**	3 heaped tbsp	trace	1	medium
Spinach and bacon salad	**451**	1 serving	9	44	medium
Spinach roulade	**327**	1 serving	16	20	high
Spinach soup, home-made	**132**	2 ladlefuls	31	trace	medium

Food	kC/ portion	Portion size	Carbs g	Fat g	Fibre
Spirali (pasta shapes), dried, boiled	**198**	1 serving	42	1	medium
Spirali, fresh, boiled	**235**	1 serving	45	2	medium
Split pea soup, canned	**142**	1 serving	24	2	high
Split ice lolly, any flavour	**83**	1 lolly	13	0	0
Sponge cake	**229**	1 slice	26	13	low
Sponge cake, fatless	**147**	1 slice	26	3	low
Sponge cake, fatless, filled with cream	**343**	1 slice	36	22	low
Sponge cake, fatless, filled with jam (conserve)	**181**	1 slice	38	3	low
Sponge cake, victoria, filled with cream	**490**	1 slice	52	31	low
Sponge cake, victoria, filled with jam (conserve)	**302**	1 slice	64	5	low
Sponge (lady) fingers	**40**	1 finger	6	1	low
Sporties, dry	**89**	25 g/1 oz/½ cup	19	trace	high
Sporties, with semi-skimmed milk	**203**	5 heaped tbsp	37	3	high
Sporties, with skimmed milk	**187**	5 heaped tbsp	37	1	high
Spotted dick	**350**	1 serving	52	16	medium
Sprats, fried (sautéed)	**393**	5 fish	4	35	low

Food	kC/ portion	Portion size	Carbs g	Fat g	Fibre
Spring greens (collard greens), steamed or boiled	20	3 heaped tbsp	2	1	medium
Spring onions (scallions)	3	1 onion	trace	trace	low
Spring roll, large	217	1 large roll	21	12	low
Spring roll, small	70	1 small roll	7	3	low
Spring vegetable soup, canned	62	2 ladlefuls	13	trace	medium
Spring vegetable soup, packet	80	2 ladlefuls	9	4	low
Sprite	85	1 tumbler	22	0	0
Sprite, diet	5	1 tumbler	0	0	0
Squab, roast	303	1 bird	0	18	0
Squab pie	470	1 serving	21	28	medium
Squash See Marrow					
Squash, butternut	9	½ medium squash	2	trace	low
Squash, fruit, diluted See individual flavours, e.g. Orange squash					
Squid, stewed in olive oil	336	1 serving	0	31	0
Squid, stuffed	85	1 squid	4	10	low
Squid rings, fried (sautéed), in batter	235	1 serving	19	12	low
Squid risotto	369	1 serving	52	15	low

Food	kC/ portion	Portion size	Carbs g	Fat g	Fibre
Starfruit	**30**	1 fruit	7	trace	medium
Starburst sweets (candies)	**185**	1 tube	38	3	0
Start, dry	**90**	25 g/1 oz/½ cup	20	trace	medium
Start, with semi-skimmed milk	**201**	5 heaped tbsp	38	3	medium
Start, with skimmed milk	**185**	5 heaped tbsp	38	1	medium
Steak, fillet, fried (sautéed)	**359**	1 fillet	0	21	0
Steak, fillet, grilled (broiled)	**336**	1 fillet	0	16	0
Steak, rump or sirloin, fried	**430**	1 steak	0	25	0
Steak, rump or sirloin, grilled	**381**	1 steak	0	21	0
Steak and kidney pie	**500**	1 serving	28	32	medium
Steak and kidney pie, individual	**484**	1 pie	38	31	medium
Steak and kidney pudding	**431**	1 serving	24	23	low
Steak and onions	**463**	1 steak	8	27	medium
Steak au poivre	**455**	1 steak	1	29	0
Steak chasseur	**417**	1 steak	7	21	0
Steak diane	**488**	1 steak	3	28	low
Steak sandwiches	**685**	1 round	34	38	low
Steamed sponge pudding	**340**	1 serving	45	16	medium
Steamed suet pudding	**221**	1 serving	34	12	low
Stem lettuce See Chinese leaves					

Food	kC/ portion	Portion size	Carbs g	Fat g	Fibre
Sticky toffee pudding	313	1 serving	47	12	low
Stifado	565	1 serving	6	16	medium
Stilton cheese, blue	103	1 small wedge	trace	9	0
Stilton cheese, white	94	1 small wedge	trace	8	0
Stock cube, chicken	32	1 cube	3	2	0
Stock cube, meat	32	1 cube	2	2	0
Stock cube, vegetable	33	1 cube	3	2	0
Stollen	177	1 slice	26	13	medium
Stout	117	1 small	6	trace	0
Straw mushrooms, canned, drained	7	¼ medium can	1	trace	0
Strawberries	27	3 heaped tbsp	6	trace	medium
Strawberries, canned in natural juice	48	3 heaped tbsp	13	trace	medium
Strawberries, canned in syrup	65	3 heaped tbsp	17	trace	medium
Strawberry cheesecake	296	1 slice	32	17	low
Strawberry dessert	101	1 small pot	16	3	0
Strawberry ice cream	89	1 scoop	12	4	0
Strawberry jam (conserve)	39	1 tbsp	10	0	0
Strawberry milkshake, made with granules and semi-skimmed milk	138	1 tumbler	23	3	low

Food	kCl/ portion	Portion size	Carbs g	Fat g	Fibre
Strawberry mousse	137	1 serving	18	6	low
Strawberry pavlova	320	1 serving	45	14	medium
Strawberry shortcake	265	1 serving	35	12	low
Strawberry sorbet	57	1 scoop	19	trace	low
Strawberry soufflé	325	1 serving	21	41	low
Streusel cake	157	1 slice	35	1	low
Striped bass, grilled (broiled)	153	1 piece of fillet	0	4	0
Stufato (Italian beef stew)	565	1 serving	6	16	medium
Stuffing, made with breadcrumbs and herbs	14	1 tbsp	3	trace	low
Stuffing, made with rice	31	1 tbsp	5	1	low
Sugar puffs, dry	97	25 g/1 oz/½ cup	22	trace	low
Sugar puffs, with semi-skimmed milk	212	5 heaped tbsp	41	2	low
Sugar puffs, with skimmed milk	196	5 heaped tbsp	41	trace	low
Sugar snap peas	57	10 pods	8	1	high
Sugar snap peas, steamed or boiled	52	3 heaped tbsp	7	1	high
Sugar, all types	20	1 tsp	5	trace	0
Sukiyaki	246	1 serving	20	9	high
Sultana bran, dry	80	25 g/1 oz/½ cup	16	trace	high

Food	kCl/portion	Portion size	Carbs g	Fat g	Fibre
Sultana bran, with semi-skimmed milk	185	5 heaped tbsp	33	3	high
Sultana bran, with skimmed milk	169	5 heaped tbsp	33	1	high
Sultana (golden raisin) cake	180	1 slice	29	6	medium
Sultanas (golden raisins)	41	1 small handful	10	trace	high
Summer pudding	266	1 serving	59	1	high
Sunflower seeds	87	1 tbsp	2	7	high
Supernoodles, all flavours	523 (avge)	1 packet	67	24	high
Surf 'n' turf	516	1 steak plus 2 breaded prawns (shrimp)	17	32	low
Sushi, mixed, average	40	1 piece	8	1	low
Sussex pond pudding	391	1 serving	50	24	low
Sustain, dry	90	25 g/1 oz/½ cup	18	1	medium
Sustain, with semi-skimmed milk	201	5 heaped tbsp	36	3	medium
Sustain, with skimmed milk	185	5 heaped tbsp	36	1	medium
Swede (rutabaga), steamed or boiled	11	3 heaped tbsp	2	trace	low
Sweet and sour chicken	165	1 serving	32	2	high
Sweet and sour pork	303	1 serving	31	9	medium

Food	kC/ portion	Portion size	Carbs g	Fat g	Fibre
Sweet and sour sauce	112	5 tbsp	trace	low	
Sweet potatoes, roasted	190	4 pieces	20	12	medium
Sweet potatoes, steamed or boiled, mashed	84	3 heaped tbsp	20	trace	medium
Sweetcorn (corn), kernels, canned	122	3 heaped tbsp	27	1	medium
Sweetcorn, on the cob	99	1 cob	17	2	medium
See also Corn cobs *and* Corn on the cob					
Swiss chard, steamed or boiled	25	3 heaped tbsp	4	trace	medium
Swiss cheese *See also* Emmental *and* Gruyère	107	1 small wedge	1	8	0
Swiss cheese fondue	492	1 serving	8	29	0
Swiss cheese fondue, with French bread	762	1 serving plus 10 cubes of bread	62	31	medium
Swiss (jelly) roll, chocolate	85	1 individual roll	14	3	low
Swiss roll, with jam (conserve)	105	1 individual roll	24	1	low
Swiss-style muesli *See* Muesli					
Swordfish steak, fried (sautéed)	294	1 steak	0	14	0

Food	kC/ portion	Portion size	Carbs g	Fat g	Fibre
Swordfish steak, grilled (broiled)	**271**	1 steak	0	9	0
Syllabub	**428**	1 serving	5	35	0
Syrup, golden (light corn)	**45**	1 tbsp	12	0	0
Syrup sauce, for ice cream, bottled, all flavours	**92** (avge)	2 tbsp	23	0	0
Syrup sponge pudding	**369**	1 serving	53	16	medium
Syrup tart	**368**	1 slice	60	14	medium

Food	kC/ portion	Portion size	Carbs g	Fat g	Fibre
Tabbouleh	**278**	3 heaped tbsp	41	10	high
Taco shell	**57**	1 shell	6	3	low
Taco shell, filled with chilli and salad	**170**	1 shell	12	10	medium
Tagliarini (pasta strands), dried, boiled	**239**	1 serving	51	2	medium
Tagliarini, fresh, boiled	**301**	1 serving	57	2	medium
Tagliatelle (pasta ribbons), dried, boiled	**239**	1 serving	51	2	medium
Tagliatelle, fresh, boiled	**301**	1 serving	57	2	medium
Tahini paste	**91**	1 tbsp	trace	9	medium
Tandoori chicken	**750**	½ small chicken	7	38	low
Tangerine	**44**	1 fruit	11	trace	medium
Tangle twister ice lolly	**90**	1 lolly	18	2	low
Tango, lemon	**98**	1 tumbler	23	trace	0
See also Apple tango, etc.					
Tango, orange	**92**	1 tumbler	25	0	0
Tapioca pudding, canned	**169**	½ large can	27	5	low
Tapioca pudding, made with semi-skimmed milk	**150**	1 serving	29	2	low
Tapioca pudding, made with skimmed milk	**134**	1 serving	29	trace	low

Food	kCl/ portion	Portion size	Carbs g	Fat g	Fibre
Taramasalata	**223**	2 tbsp	2	23	low
Tartare sauce	**43**	1 tbsp	3	3	low
Taxi chocolate bar	**134**	1 standard bar	17	7	low
Tea, black	**0**	1 cup	trace	trace	0
Tea, with lemon	**0**	1 cup	trace	trace	0
Tea, with lemon and sugar	**20**	1 cup plus 1 spoonful of sugar	5	trace	0
Tea, with milk	**7**	1 cup	trace	1	0
Teacake	**180**	1 individual teacake	32	4	low
Teacake, toasted, with butter	**254**	1 individual teacake	32	12	low
Teacake, toasted, with low-fat spread	**219**	1 individual teacake	32	8	low
Tempura	**328**	1 serving	40	8	low
Tequila	**55**	1 single measure	trace	0	0
Tequila sunrise	**232**	1 cocktail	24	trace	0
Teriyaki sauce	**14**	1 tbsp	3	trace	low
Thai chicken, with noodles	**506**	1 serving	59	15	high
Thai chicken soup	**111**	2 ladlefuls	21	1	low
Thai fragrant rice, steamed or boiled	**248**	1 serving	56	2	low
Thai green chicken curry	**331**	1 serving	6	23	low
Thai red beef curry	**602**	1 serving	6	49	low

Food	kC/ portion	Portion size	Carbs g	Fat g	Fibre
Thousand island dressing	**59**	1 tbsp	2	5	low
Thousand island dressing, low-calorie	**12**	1 tbsp	1	1	low
Tia maria	**79**	1 single measure	6	0	0
Tilsit cheese	**96**	1 small wedge	trace	7	0
Time out chocolate bar	**105**	1 finger	6	6	low
Tip top topping	**16**	1 tbsp	1	1	low
Tipsy cake	**488**	1 slice	41	32	low
Tiramisu	**222**	1 serving	24	11	low
Tisanes, all flavours	**0**	1 cup	trace	trace	0
Tizer	**82**	1 tumbler	20	trace	low
Tizer, diet	**0**	1 tumbler	trace	trace	low
Toad-in-the-hole	**462**	2 thick sausages plus batter	33	30	medium
Toast, white, with butter	**155**	1 medium slice	18	9	low
Toast, white, with low-fat spread	**120**	1 medium slice	18	5	low
Toast, wholemeal, with butter	**153**	1 medium slice	15	10	high
Toast, wholemeal, with low-fat spread	**118**	1 medium slice	15	6	high
Toasted cheese and ham sandwiches	**438**	1 round	36	27	medium
Toffee bon bons	**29**	1 toffee	6	1	0

Food	kCl/ portion	Portion size	Carbs g	Fat g	Fibre
Toffee apple	**251**	1 apple	66	trace	high
Toffee crisp chocolate bar	**237**	1 standard bar	30	12	low
Toffee fudge ice cream	**90**	1 scoop	12	4	0
Toffees, mixed	**20**	1 toffee	1	0	0
Toffos, assorted	**203**	1 tube	31	8	0
Tofu, firm	**62**	½ block	2	2	low
Tofu, fried (sautéed)	**308**	½ block	12	24	medium
Tofu, marinated, baked	**139**	½ block	4	10	medium
Tofu, silken	**55**	½ block	2	2	low
Tofu, smoked	**148**	½ block	1	9	low
Tofu and vegetable stir-fry	**334**	1 serving	24	21	high
Tofu burger	**154**	1 burger	6	12	medium
Tomato	**13**	1 fruit	2	trace	low
Tomato, stuffed, baked	**53**	1 large	9	1	medium
Tomato and herb pasta sauce, ready-made	**79**	¼ jar	16	trace	low
Tomato and lentil soup, canned	**108**	2 ladlefuls	20	trace	medium
Tomato and lentil soup, home-made	**188**	2 ladlefuls	26	8	medium
Tomato and lentil soup, instant	**73**	1 mug	15	1	low
Tomato and onion salad	**35**	1 serving	11	trace	medium

Food	kCl/portion	Portion size	Carbs g	Fat g	Fibre
Tomato and onion salad, dressed	132	1 serving	11	17	medium
Tomato and orange soup, canned	80	2 ladlefuls	17	1	low
Tomato and orange soup, home-made	103	2 ladlefuls	15	4	medium
Tomato and rice soup, canned	94	2 ladlefuls	17	2	low
Tomato chutney	24	1 tbsp	6	trace	low
Tomato juice	28	1 tumbler	6	trace	low
Tomato juice cocktail	36	1 tumbler	19	0	low
Tomato ketchup (catsup)	15	1 tbsp	4	trace	low
Tomato relish	16	1 tbsp	3	trace	low
Tomato risotto	403	1 serving	58	18	medium
Tomato sauce, home-made	67	5 tbsp	6	4	medium
Tomato soup, cream of, canned	110	2 ladlefuls	12	7	low
Tomato soup, home-made	86	2 ladlefuls	11	4	low
Tomato soup, instant	85	1 mug	17	2	medium
Tomato soup, low-fat, canned	50	2 ladlefuls	8	1	low
Tomatoes, canned	32	1 small can	6	trace	medium
Tomatoes, fried (sautéed)	68	2 halves	4	6	low
Tomatoes, grilled (broiled)	37	2 halves1	7	1	low
Tomatoes, sieved	29	5 tbsp	6	trace	0

Food	kCl/portion	Portion size	Carbs g	Fat g	Fibre
Tomatoes, stewed	25	2 whole	4	trace	medium
Tomatoes, sun-dried	5	1 piece	1	trace	low
Tomatoes, sun-dried, in oil, drained	7	1 piece	1	1	low
Tongue, lunch	43	1 slice	0	3	0
Tongue, ox, pressed and sliced	73	1 slice	0	6	0
Tongue, pork, pressed and sliced	47	1 slice	0	4	0
Tongues, lambs', canned	213	½ medium can	0	16	0
Tonic water	43	1 tumbler	10	0	0
Tonic water, low-calorie	4	1 tumbler	0	0	0
Topic chocolate bar	233	1 standard bar	27	12	low
Tornado ice cream	61	1 ice	15	0	0
Tortellini (stuffed pasta), dried, boiled	291	1 serving	45	6	medium
Tortellini, fresh, boiled	229	1 serving	40	4	medium
Tortilla (spanish omelette)	328	2 eggs	17	22	medium
Tortilla chips, all flavours	229	1 small bag	30	11	medium
Tortillas, corn	58	1 medium tortilla	12	1	medium
Tortillas, flour	159	1 medium tortilla	27	3	medium
Tournedos rossini	477	1 fillet steak	9	25	low

Food	kCl/portion	Portion size	Carbs g	Fat g	Fibre
Tracker bars, all flavours	**192** (avge)	1 standard bar	22	10	medium
Treacle, black (molasses)	**38**	1 tbsp	10	0	0
Treacle pudding	**369**	1 serving	53	16	medium
Treacle tart	**368**	1 slice	60	14	medium
Treacle toffee	**20**	1 piece	1	0	0
Trifle	**372**	1 serving	69	6	high
Trinity cream	**453**	1 serving	15	50	0
Trio chocolate bar	**111**	1 standard bar	12	6	low
Triple chocolate bar	**99**	1 standard bar	12	5	low
Tropical fruit salad	**86**	3 heaped tbsp	22	trace	medium
Trout, baked, stuffed	**326**	1 medium fish	41	39	medium
Trout, fried (sautéed)	**232**	1 medium fish	0	13	0
Trout, grilled (broiled)	**209**	1 medium fish	0	8	0
Trout, poached or steamed	**200**	1 medium fish	0	7	0
Trout, smoked	**136**	1 fillet	0	5	0
Trout, smoked, pâté	**269**	1 serving	0	24	0
Trout meunière	**388**	1 medium fish	trace	29	0
Trout with almonds	**464**	1 medium fish	1	36	medium
Truffles, chocolate	**50**	1 truffle	6	2	low
Truite au bleu	**200**	1 medium fish	0	7	0

Food	kCl portion	Portion size	Carbs g	Fat g	Fibre
Tuc crackers	**25**	1 cracker	3	1	low
Tuc savoury sandwiches	**76**	1 sandwich	7	5	low
Tuna, canned in brine, drained	**107**	½ standard can	0	trace	0
Tuna, canned in oil, drained	**182**	½ standard can	0	7	0
Tuna and cucumber sandwiches	**352**	1 round	35	18	medium
Tuna and pasta casserole	**285**	1 serving	30	9	medium
Tuna and sweetcorn pasta	**451**	1 serving	50	11	medium
Tuna mornay	**241**	1 serving	7	10	low
Tuna mousse	**185**	1 serving	6	10	low
Tuna salad	**138**	1 serving	5	1	high
Tuna salad, with mayonnaise	**344**	1 serving	11	23	high
Tuna steak, fried (sautéed)	**345**	1 steak	0	15	0
Tuna steak, grilled (broiled)	**322**	1 steak	0	10	0
Tunes sweets (candies)	**145**	1 tube	36	0	0
Turbot, grilled (broiled)	**194**	1 piece of fillet	0	6	0
Turbot, steamed or poached	**159**	1 piece of fillet	0	1	0
Turkey, breast, smoked	**21**	1 slice	trace	trace	0
Turkey, fillets, fried (sautéed)	**248**	1 medium fillet	0	9	0
Turkey fillets, grilled (broiled)	**225**	1 medium fillet	0	4	0

Food	kC/ portion	Portion size	Carbs g	Fat g	Fibre
Turkey fillets, fried, in breadcrumbs	326	1 medium fillet	13	9	low
Turkey, minced (ground), stewed	197	1 serving	0	5	0
Turkey, roast, with skin	171	2 medium slices	0	6	0
Turkey, roast, without skin	140	2 medium slices	0	3	0
Turkey, roast, with stuffing and sausagemeat	229	1 serving	12	5	medium
Turkey and vegetable casserole	298	1 serving	32	8	medium
Turkey and vegetable soup, home-made	134	2 ladlefuls	14	4	medium
Turkey and vegetable stir-fry	259	1 serving	31	3	high
Turkey bacon, grilled (broiled)	34	1 slice	trace	3	0
Turkey burger in a bun, with relish, home-made	357	1 burger in a bun	32	9	low
Turkey fingers, fried (sautéed), in batter orbreadcrumbs	178	1 finger	11	11	low
Turkey ham	36	1 slice	trace	1	0
Turkey pot pie	485	1 slice	28	39	low
Turkey roll	41	1 slice	trace	2	0
Turkey sandwiches	345	1 round	34	19	medium
Turkey soup, home-made	111	2 ladlefuls	7	2	0

Food	kCl portion	Portion size	Carbs g	Fat g	Fibre
Turkey stew	**430**	1 serving	65	3	medium
Turkish delight, chocolate covered-	**185**	1 standard bar	37	4	0
Turkish delight, in icing (confectioners') sugar	**29**	1 cube	8	0	0
Turnips, glazed	**55**	3 heaped tbsp	15	trace	medium
Turnips, steamed or boiled	**12**	3 heaped tbsp	2	trace	medium
Tuscan bean salad	**120**	3 heaped tbsp	12	5	high
Tutti frutti ice cream	**75**	1 scoop	5	7	low
Twiglets	**136**	1 small bag	16	3	medium
Twirl chocolate bar	**115**	1 finger	12	7	0
Twistetti (pasta shapes), dried, boiled	**198**	1 serving	42	1	medium
Twistetti, fresh, boiled	**235**	1 serving	45	2	medium
Twix chocolate bar	**143**	1 finger	18	7	low
Twix ice cream	**228**	1 standard bar	23	14	low
Tzatziki	**20**	2 tbsp	1	1	low

Food	kC/portion	Portion size	Carbs g	Fat g	Fibre
Vacherin, with cream and fruit	**320**	1 slice	45	14	medium
Vanilla fudge	**77**	1 square	14	2	0
Vanilla cheesecake	**490**	1 slice	30	27	low
Vanilla ice cream, dairy	**97**	1 scoop	12	5	0
Vanilla ice cream, non-dairy	**89**	1 scoop	11	4	0
Vanilla soufflé	**236**	1 serving	26	1	low
Veal, cutlet, fried (sautéed), in breadcrumbs,	**376**	1 cutlet	8	14	low
Veal, cutlet, grilled (broiled)	**300**	1 cutlet	0	9	0
Veal, escalope, fried, in breadcrumbs	**335**	1 escalope	20	15	low
Veal, roast	**230**	2 thick slices	0	11	0
Veal birds	**450**	2 rolls	12	20	low
Veal fricassée	**339**	1 serving	34	9	low
Vegemite	**8**	1 tsp	trace	0	0
Vegetable bake	**360**	1 serving	33	10	high
Vegetable casserole	**228**	1 serving	33	6	high
Vegetable cottage pie	**350**	1 serving	48	12	high
Vegetable curry	**183**	1 serving	34	4	high
Vegetable deluxe burger	**423**	1 burger in a bun	54	18	high
Vegetable goulash	**338**	1 serving	142	15	high

Food	kC/portion	Portion size	Carbs g	Fat g	Fibre
Vegetable juice	41	1 tumbler	9	trace	low
Vegetable lasagne	424	1 serving	50	10	high
Vegetable pâté	138	1 serving	1	10	low
Vegetable pie	425	1 individual pie	52	23	medium
Vegetable risotto	372	1 serving	58	15	low
Vegetable samosa	236	1 samosa	11	21	medium
Vegetable soup, canned	74	2 ladlefuls	13	1	high
Vegetable soup, home-made	93	2 ladlefuls	4	trace	high
Vegetable soup, packet	46	2 ladlefuls	8	1	low
Vegetable stew	186	1 serving	31	4	high
Vegetable stir-fry	169	1 serving7	15	6	high
Vegetable terrine	155	1 thick slice	17	7	high
Vegetables, mixed, canned, drained	38	3 heaped tbsp	6	1	medium
Vegetables, mixed, frozen, cooked	42	3 heaped tbsp	7	trace	high
Veggie burger	85	1 burger	5	4	medium
Veggie sausage	75	1 sausage	6	4	medium
Velouté sauce	99	5 tbsp	4	9	low
Venison, roast	198	2 thick slices	0	6	0
Venison, stewed	225	1 serving	8	7	low

Food	kCl/ portion	Portion size	Carbs g	Fat g	Fibre
Vermicelli (pasta strands), dried, boiled	239	1 serving	51	2	medium
Vermicelli, fresh, boiled	301	1 serving	57	2	medium
Vermouth, bianco	67	1 double measure	8	0	0
Vermouth, extra dry	59	1 double measure	3	0	0
Vermouth, red	75	1 double measure	8	0	0
Vermouth, rosso	85	1 double measure	8	0	0
Vichyssoise, canned	108	2 ladlefuls	12	6	low
Vichyssoise, home-made	117	2 ladlefuls	8	6	low
Victoria sandwich, filled with jam (conserve)	302	1 slice	64	5	low
Viennetta, all flavours	227 (avge)	1 slice	23	14	0
Vienna bread	109	1 thick slice	15	1	low
Viennese finger, filled	81	1 biscuit (cookie)	9	5	low
Vimto	52	1 tumbler	20	trace	0
Vinaigrette dressing	101	1 tbsp	trace	11	0
Vinaigrette dressing, low-calorie	5	1 tbsp	1	trace	0
Vine leaves, stuffed	221	2 rolls	19	9	high
Vinegar, all types	1	1 tsp	0	0	0
Vitbe bread	82	1 medium slice	16	1	medium

Food	kC/ portion	Portion size	Carbs g	Fat g	Fibre
Vitello tonnato	**594**	1 escalope	20	37	low
Vodka	**55**	1 single measure	trace	0	0
Vodka and orange	**108**	1 single measure	7	0	0
Vodka and tonic	**76**	1 single measure plus 1 mixer	5	0	0
Vodka and tonic, low-calorie	**58**	1 single measure plus 1 mixer	trace	trace	0
Vodka martini	**114**	1 cocktail	3	trace	0
Vol-au-vents, all flavours	**286** (avge)	1 medium	20	18	low
Vol-au-vents, cocktail, all flavours	**143** (avge)	1 small	10	9	low

Food	kC/ portion	Portion size	Carbs g	Fat g	Fibre
Wafer biscuits (cookies), chocolate-covered	**115**	1 biscuit	13	6	low
Wafer biscuits, filled	**39**	1 biscuit	7	2	low
Wafers, for ice cream	**17**	1 wafer	4	trace	low
Waffle, potato, fried (sautéed) or baked	**84**	1 waffle	13	3	low
Waffle, sweet	**240**	1 waffle	30	8	low
Waffles, sweet, with maple syrup	**533**	2 waffles	75	16	medium
Waffles, with bacon and maple syrup	**799**	2 waffles plus 2 rashers (slices) of bacon	75	48	medium
Walnut cake	**344**	1 slice	34	19	medium
Walnut whip	**165**	1 whip	20	8	low
Walnut whirl, chocolate	**20**	1 chocolate	2	1	low
Walnuts, shelled	**172**	25 g/1 oz/¼ cup	1	17	high
Water biscuits (crackers)	**33**	1 biscuit	6	1	low
Water chestnuts, canned, drained	**14**	4 pieces	3	trace	low
Watercress	**3**	1 good handful	trace	trace	medium
Watercress soup	**99**	2 ladlefuls	14	2	low
Watermelon	**66**	1 large wedge	14	1	low

Food	kCl/ portion	Portion size	Carbs g	Fat g	Fibre
Weetabix, dry	**64**	1 biscuit	13	trace	high
Weetabix, with semi-skimmed milk	**169**	2 biscuits	32	trace	high
Weetabix, with skimmed milk	**185**	2 biscuits	32	2	high
Weetaflakes, dry	**90**	25 g/1 oz/½ cup	20	1	high
Weetaflakes, with semi skimmed milk-	**201**	5 heaped tbsp	38	3	high
Weetaflakes, with skimmed milk	**185**	5 heaped tbsp	38	1	high
Weetos, dry	**96**	25 g/1 oz/½ cup	20	1	medium
Weetos, with semi-skimmed milk	**172**	5 heaped tbsp	30	4	medium
Weetos, with skimmed milk	**154**	5 heaped tbsp	30	2	medium
Welsh rarebit	**242**	1 slice	21	13	low
Wensleydale cheese	**94**	1 small wedge	trace	8	0
Westphalian ham	**29**	1 slice	trace	2	0
Wheat bran	**31**	1 tbsp	4	1	high
Wheat crunchies, all flavours	**180** (avge)	1 small packet	20	9	low
Whelks, boiled	**14**	1 serving	trace	trace	0
Whippy ice cream	**85**	1 cornet	12	3	low
Whisky	**55**	1 single measure	trace	0	0

Food	kC/ portion	Portion size	Carbs g	Fat g	Fibre
Whisky and coke	**99**	1 single measure plus 1 mixer	6	0	0
Whisky and coke, low-calorie	**56**	1 single measure plus 1 mixer	trace	trace	0
Whisky and ginger ale	**75**	1 single measure plus 1 mixer	5	0	0
Whisky and ginger ale, low-calorie	**55**	1 single measure plus 1 tumbler	trace	0	0
Whisky mac	**255**	1 single measure plus 1 double measure	trace	0	0
Whisky sour	**157**	1 cocktail	14	0	0
White pudding, fried (sautéed) or baked	**450**	2 thick slices	36	32	low
White sauce, savoury, made with semi-skimmed milk	**96**	5 tbsp	8	6	low
White sauce, savoury, made with skimmed milk	**86**	5 tbsp	8	5	low
White sauce, sweet, made with semi-skimmed milk	**112**	5 tbsp	14	5	low
White sauce, sweet, made with skimmed milk	**92**	5 tbsp	14	4	low
White stilton cheese	**94**	1 small wedge	trace	8	0
White wine sauce	**75**	5 tbsp	6	2	low

Food	kCl/portion	Portion size	Carbs g	Fat g	Fibre
Whitebait, fried (sautéed)	**525**	1 serving	5	47	low
Whiting, fried (sautéed), in breadcrumbs	**334**	1 fillet	12	17	low
Whiting, poached or steamed	**110**	1 fillet	0	1	0
Whiting, smoked, poached	**166**	1 fillet	1	1	0
Wholegrain mustard	**7**	1 tsp	1	trace	low
Wholenut chocolate bar	**270**	1 standard bar	24	17	medium
Whopper	**660**	1 burger	47	40	high
Whopper, with cheese	**760**	1 burger	47	48	high
Whopper, double	**920**	2 burgers	47	21	high
Whopper, double, with cheese	**1010**	2 burgers	47	67	high
Wiener schnitzel	**335**	1 schnitzel	20	15	low
Wild rice, cooked	**182**	1 serving	6	trace	0
Wild rice mix, cooked	**177**	1 serving	31	1	low
Winders, real fruit	**55**	1 roll	11	1	low
Wine gums	**119**	1 tube	27	trace	0
Wine, dry white, sparkling	**95**	1 wine glass	2	0	0
Wine, dry white	**82**	1 wine glass	1	0	0
Wine, low-alcohol, red	**70**	1 wine glass	2	0	0
Wine, low-alcohol, rosé	**70**	1 wine glass	2	0	0
Wine, low-alcohol, white	**70**	1 wine glass	2	0	0

Food	kC/ portion	Portion size	Carbs g	Fat g	Fibre
Wine, medium white	94	1 wine glass	4	0	0
Wine, mulled	105	1 wine glass	5	0	0
Wine, red	85	1 wine glass	trace	trace	0
Wine, rosé	89	1 wine glass	1	0	0
Wine, sweet	117	1 wine glass	7	0	0
Winkles	14	1 serving	trace	trace	low
Winter radish	12	1 radish	2	trace	0
Wispa chocolate bar	210	1 standard bar	21	13	0
Wispa, gold	265	1 standard bar	29	15	0
Wispa, mint	275	1 standard bar	27	17	0
Witch, fried (sautéed), in breadcrumbs	342	1 medium fish	15	21	low
Witch, grilled (broiled)	158	1 medium fish	0	4	0
Witch, poached or steamed	112	1 medium fish	0	1	0
Woodcock, roast	303	1 bird	0	18	0
Worcestershire sauce	17	1 tbsp	4	0	0
Wotsits, all flavours	115 (avge)	1 small packet	12	7	low

Food	kC/portion	Portion size	Carbs g	Fat g	Fibre

Food	kC/ portion	Portion size	Carbs g	Fat g	Fibre
Yam, roast	**156**	4 pieces	33	5	medium
Yam, steamed or boiled, mashed	**133**	3 heaped tbsp	33	trace	medium
Yeast extract	**9**	1 tsp	trace	trace	0
Yellow bean sauce	**19**	1 tbsp	4	trace	low
Yellow beans, fresh, steamed or boiled	**25**	3 heaped tbsp	5	trace	high
Yellow melon	**63**	1 large wedge	15	trace	medium
Yoghurt (plain)	**99**	1 individual pot	10	4	0
Yoghurt, all flavours	**131** (avge)	1 individual pot	20	4	0
Yoghurt, bio	**56**	1 small pot	7	1	0
Yoghurt, custard-style	**161**	1 small pot	3	13	0
Yoghurt, drinking	**124**	1 tumbler	26	trace	0
Yoghurt, fruit corner	**219**	1 individual carton	26	7	low
Yoghurt, greek-style, cows'	**161**	1 individual pot	3	13	0
Yoghurt, greek-style, sheep's	**149**	1 individual pot	8	10	0
Yoghurt, low-calorie	**51**	1 individual pot	7	trace	0
Yoghurt, low-fat, plain	**70**	1 individual pot	9	1	0
Yoghurt, low-fat, all flavours	**112** (avge)	1 individual pot	22	1	0
Yoghurt, soya	**90**	1 individual pot	5	5	0

Food	kC/portion	Portion size	Carbs g	Fat g	Fibre
Yoghurt ice-cream, all flavours	**53** (avge)	1 scoop	8	1	low
Yoghurt jelly (jello), made with plain, low-fat yoghurt	**60**	1 serving	12	1	0
Yorkie bar, milk	**317**	1 standard bar	35	18	0
Yorkie bar, nut	**312**	1 standard bar	26	10	low
Yorkie bar, raisin and biscuit (cookie)	**265**	1 standard bar	32	13	low
Yorkshire parkin	**185**	1 piece	29	7	low
Yorkshire pudding	**62**	1 small pudding	7	3	low

Food	kC/ portion	Portion size	Carbs g	Fat g	Fibre
Zabaglione	**87**	1 serving	8	3	0
Zite (pasta shapes), dried, boiled	**198**	1 serving	42	1	medium
Zite, fresh, boiled	**235**	1 serving	45	2	medium
Zoom ice lolly	**46**	1 lolly	10	trace	0
Zucchini See Courgettes					